# Praise for The Be

"A tome to be passed on to beauty-see... ...The *Beauty Witch's Secrets* is chock full of luxuriant magickal potions and elixirs, rituals and spells, and advice to enchant—and beautify—your everyday life. Reading it is like sipping champagne while soaking in a perfumed bath lined with flowers. A must-have for the most ultra-glam witches!"

> —Carolyn Turgeon, editor in chief of *Enchanted Living Magazine* and author of eight books, including *Mermaid: A Twist on the Classic Tale*

"Prepare to be enchanted: this comprehensive manual for magickal self-care, rich with intriguing potions and wise advice, is a splendid addition to any woman's beauty library—and it's also great fun to read. Alise makes me want to get out my cauldron and start stirring up these helpful, delicious-sounding beauty recipes."

> —Cait Johnson, author of *Witch in the Kitchen* and *Witch Wisdom for Magical Aging*

"Finally, a book that encompasses the true splendor of beauty's magic. This book is a seduction of the senses. Alise truly embodies the spell that beauty has the power to cast, and her innate potion of wisdom is poured onto these pages. This book and its infinite charm will leave you glowing like the full moon, head to toe, and from the inside out."

> —Mary Lofgren, author of *Sacred Seduction*, somatic coach, and founder of The School of Sensual Living™

"This enchanting book is utterly spellbinding! Alise Marie shares her gift for extracting the essence of powerful plant magic and elevating it into high art. Her unguents, lotions, and potions, along with exquisite rituals of self-care, will help every woman look—and feel—more beautiful. Alise Marie is a true beauty alchemist, and her witchy wisdom will weave its spell on you!"

> —Rona Berg, bestselling author of *Beauty: The New Basics* and *Fast Beauty*

"Every witch deserves a little me time. Alise Marie's complete plant-powered, moon-infused self-care manual seductively and lovingly reveals how to conjure your authentic glamour. This is the book Macbeth's witches sorely needed."

—Laren Stover, author of *Bohemian Manifesto*
and *The Bombshell Manual of Style*

"Alise Marie has created an enchantingly glamorous guide to beauty magic. Sharing her most bewitching mysteries, *The Beauty Witch's Secrets* showcases the magical art of creating beauty inside and out. Combining elements of self-care and otherworldly glamour, readers will learn recipes and rituals for facial and body treatments, restorative baths, magical martinis, and much more! This is a book for those seeking to live life like a total glam God/dess!"

—Michael Herkes, author of *The GLAM Witch*,
*Witchcraft for Daily Self-Care*, and *Love
Spells for the Modern Witch*

# THE
# Beauty
# Witch's
# SECRETS

# About The Author

———— ·•▶♦•◀•◆•◁— ————

Actress, writer, and certified holistic nutritionist, Alise Marie is passionate about a plant-powered lifestyle aligned with the cycles of the earth, moon and stars. She has been concocting health and beauty potions for over thirty years, drawing from ancient traditions, herbalism, astrology, tarot, and earth magick. She invites you to enjoy these seductive rituals that embrace life with glamour, sensuality, and *joie de vivre*.

Ms. Marie has been featured internationally in magazines, websites, and live events. She is a contributor to Enchanted Living magazine, which also presents her monthly online column, *The Beauty Witch*. She also appears as a contributing author in *The Unicorn Handbook* (Harper Collins, June 2020). Her line of eco-luxe beauty potions can be found on her website www.thebeautywitch.com.

# To Write to the Author

If you wish to contact the author or would like more information about this book, please write to the author in care of Llewellyn Worldwide Ltd. and we will forward your request. Both the author and publisher appreciate hearing from you and learning of your enjoyment of this book and how it has helped you. Llewellyn Worldwide Ltd. cannot guarantee that every letter written to the author can be answered, but all will be forwarded. Please write to:

Alise Marie
℅ Llewellyn Worldwide
2143 Wooddale Drive
Woodbury, MN 55125-2989

Please enclose a self-addressed stamped envelope for reply,
or $1.00 to cover costs. If outside the U.S.A., enclose
an international postal reply coupon.

Many of Llewellyn's authors have websites with additional
information and resources. For more information,
please visit our website at http://www.llewellyn.com.

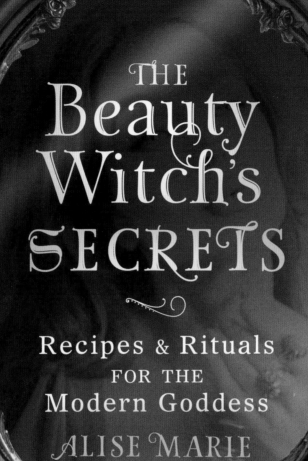

# THE
# Beauty
# Witch's
# SECRETS

## Recipes & Rituals
### FOR THE
## Modern Goddess

#### ALISE MARIE

Llewellyn Publications
Woodbury, Minnesota

FIRST EDITION
First Printing, 2022

Cover design and art direction by Shira Atakpu
Cover photo by Alise Marie
Editing by Laura Kurtz
Interior photos by Alise Marie

Llewellyn Publications is a registered trademark of Llewellyn Worldwide Ltd.

**Library of Congress Cataloging-in-Publication Data (Pending)**
ISBN: 978-0-7387-6984-4

Llewellyn Publications
A Division of Llewellyn Worldwide Ltd.
2143 Wooddale Drive
Woodbury, MN 55125-2989
www.llewellyn.com

Printed in the United States of America

For the Great Cat in the Sky,

and for the Little Moon.

# Contents

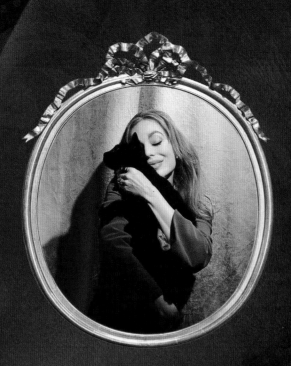

# Acknowledgments

M y most sincere gratitude to Elysia Gallo and the team at Llewellyn; Kat Neff, Karen S.Wilshinsky, Esq.; Phillip H. Farber; Carolyn Turgeon, Lisa D. Gill, and all at Enchanted Living; Paule Saviano; Rona Berg; Laren Stover; Michael Herkes; Cait Johnson; Mary Lofgren; Family, Friends, and Dear Ones; Pedro and Belilli; and most of all, to you, as you hold this book in your hands. Merci, mes chéris.

And to Jonathan Daniel Donahue, for absolutely everything. *C'est une belle histoire.*

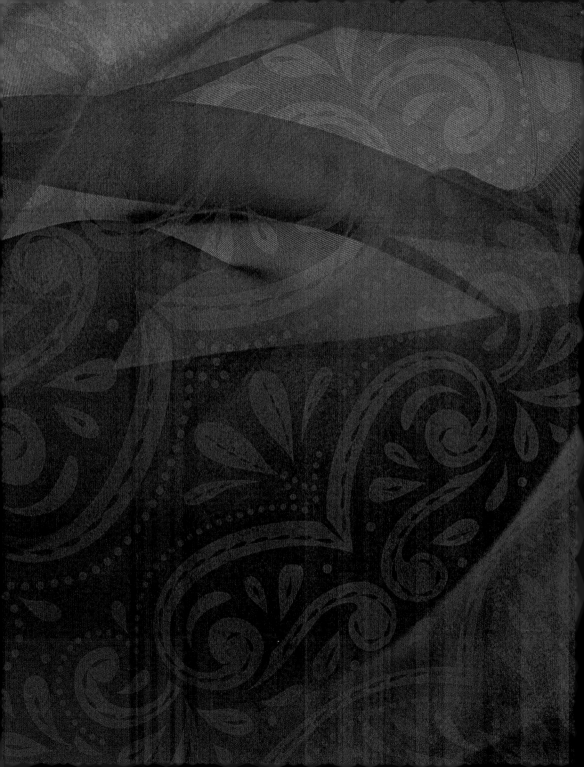

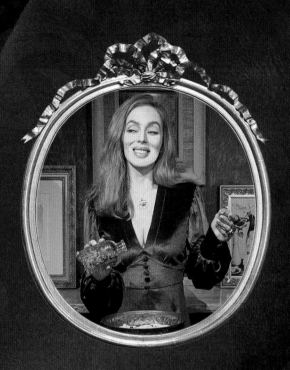

# Introduction

$\mathcal{A}$ magnificent creature appears in front of you, seemingly out of nowhere. Though you find her startling at first, you cannot take your eyes off her: she absolutely *glows*. From the top of her shimmering tresses all the way down to her silken toes, she radiates inner light, magnetic sensuality, and the confidence that comes with it. *How on earth does she get that way?* The urge to chalk it off to genetics immediately surfaces, but you quickly realize that what she possesses, what she *knows*, has little to do with such conventions. She is a Witch. With knowledge of plant magick, planetary cycles, and lunar phases in her cauldron, she concocts beauty potions that keep her at her most spellbinding, inside and out, throughout every stage of her life. Time tested, powerful, and visibly effective, her potions *work*. And she wants to share her secrets with you.

Welcome to the Lair of the Beauty Witch. Inside these velvet walls cherished secrets of spellbinding beauty are kept, nurtured, and made more powerful by time. Advertising and its false hype have no place within this enchanted realm. Here, knowledge is power. A Beauty Witch knows not only how to *awaken* her celestial beauty, but how to *reveal* it. She knows how to light the candle that glows brightly inside her, and tether it to the endless shimmer of the cosmos. Think of it as drawing starlight down from the heavens onto your body, drinking in illumination, and casting your spell upon the world. The sheer empowerment of concocting high-performance potions entwined with the heightened pleasure of anointing yourself with them creates an unstoppable force. Sauntering through each moment knowing that golden solar light shines from your eyes, your skin effortlessly reflects luminescent moonglow, and your smile captivates with millions of glittering stars, you have tapped into that power, and the confidence that comes with it.

Inside these pages you will discover the secrets for bewitching beauty, aided and abetted by practical magick. The routine of getting ready becomes instantly elevated from a monotonous chore to one of *ceremony*; sensual, empowering, and infinitely pleasurable. You are invited to align with the cycles of the moon, the stars, and the power of nature to reveal the enchanted beauty that is your birthright. Potent potions, sensual rituals, healing brews, and stylish cocktails are gathered in this book to bestow ageless beauty, seductive confidence, and a radiant celestial glow from the inside out. You will find many familiar, beloved Witch's herbs in these recipes, but you will also discover new magickal cohorts, for though traditional European herbs and flowers are undeniably effective, they often benefit from a power boost by way of treasures from faraway lands—those of even older magickal practices. And though they may take a bit more effort to procure, the results are entirely worth it! Where to procure? Not to worry, *mes chéris*, you will find a complete list of reliable online shops in the Resources section (p. 235). Imagine hair so soft and silky that it invites a lover's touch, skin that beckons gentle caresses, and a scent so alluring that it not only attracts, but also inspires. Deep inside you lies a creature of unstoppable force. All you have to do is reclaim her. I'll let you in on a secret: age and cheekbones have nothing to do with it. Nor does body type. Beauty is your *birthright*. It is not vain—it is a primal awareness of how to care for yourself, and the understanding that you are worth it.

This is where beauty magick comes in. I use the spelling of the word *magick* here and throughout this book, as by definition it means the art of utilizing natural forces to bring about change. Potions born of high-vibration ingredients, created with intent, and bathed beneath the heavens carry just that kind of charge. This is not to be confused with advanced ritual magicks, the kind that are only to be practiced by the most experienced Witch, but rather a very benevolent form of practical magick that can be utilized by everyone. Its only design is to build inner strength which then extends outward to the physical. As with all embodiments of ancient wisdom, it must be performed with integrity. And I say it's high time we bring it out of the broom closet and into the spotlight.

Long before this book was completed, I was dreaming up its title. As intuition often does, it spoke to me quietly, but with purpose: *The Beauty Witch*. I spoke the words aloud, and kept on repeating them as they grew, from a tiny sparkle into bright swathes of voluptuous color that filled the room. I was ecstatic. I knew this was not just my book title, but a moniker that perfectly illustrated a lifestyle I was fervent to share. I searched to see if it existed anywhere, and found something most interesting: The term *beauty witch* had been coined in Asia under a rather superstitious influence. The story went that if a woman of a certain age (or well past) looked youthful, it meant that she must be having some serious "work" done. Glowing skin, sumptuous hair, and a vibrant, supple body couldn't possibly occur *naturally* past a certain brief point in our lives, therefore some kind of witchcraft must be involved.

Now this line of reasoning isn't entirely false. We can indeed fall prey to the body's inclination to age poorly, and often prematurely, if we aren't paying attention. But Smart Witches know better. With a glorious, plant-powered cauldron of wisdom just waiting to be had, why, at any age, would we settle for being anything less than our most bewitching?

It's as liberating as dancing naked in the rain to know that you can infuse magick into every cell of your being. By aligning with natural forces, we take back our elemental connection to the cycles of the earth, the seasons, the movements of the planets, and the phases of the moon. No longer are we beholden to chemically laden commercial products, smarmy marketing campaigns, or invasive procedures. We know how to concoct potions that *work*. Whether you are a maiden still battling teenage acne, a mother trying to balance hormones *and* a family, or a crone goddess disinterested in aging *anything* less than gracefully, you will find potent natural solutions in these pages.

The moment is here to open up to the gifts that the stars, earth, and sea offer us. To embrace our power. And to be our most beautiful, inside and out. Won't you join me?

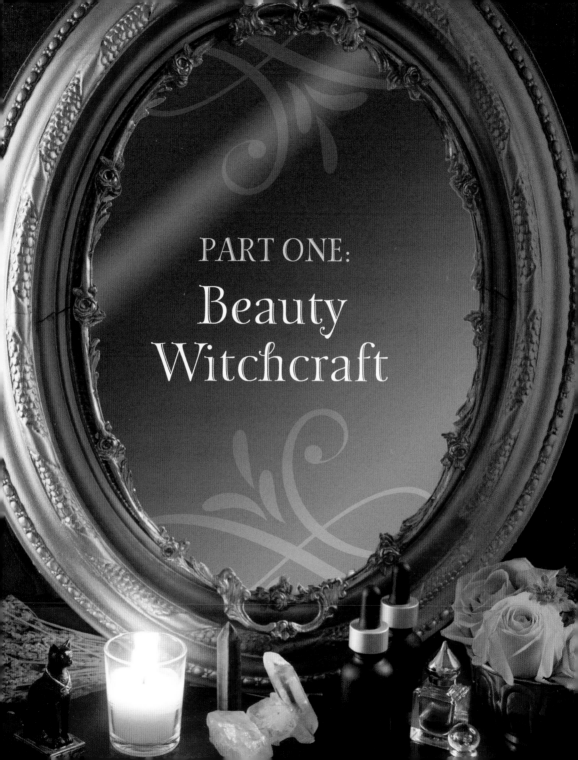

# PART ONE:
# Beauty Witchcraft

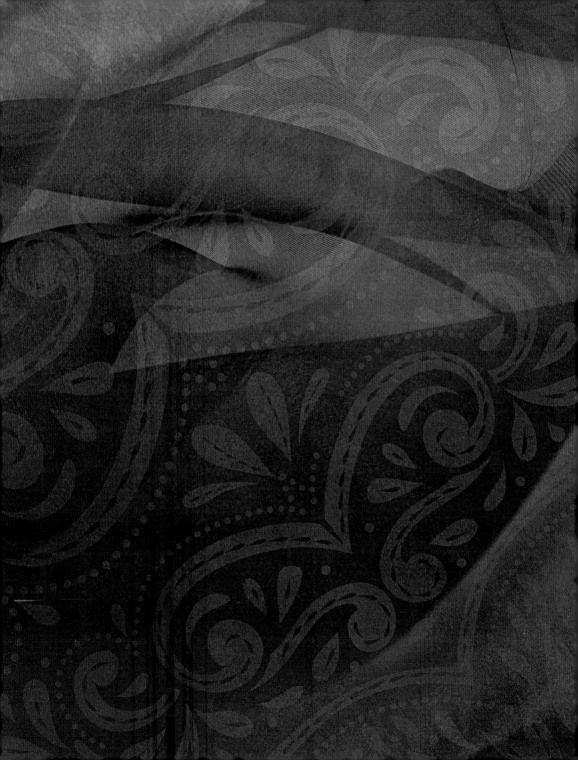

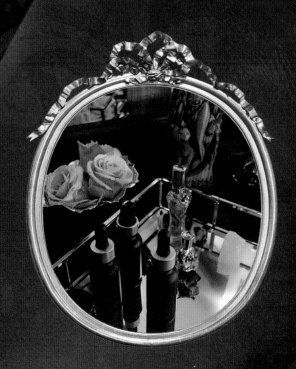

### Chapter One

# Ritual and Your Altar

itual. The word alone conjures the most sublime images. Those sacred moments spent in timeless, otherworldly reverie. The passions that give rise to taking control of our state of affairs. We use ritual only for the greatest good, utilizing the highest vibration and the most acute wisdom as we send our wishes out into the world. Manipulation is not tolerated by Smart Witches, nor is the disregard of cosmic timing. Just because you *want* something, doesn't mean it is meant to be. Karmas govern everything, *mes amours*, so pay close attention. Smart Witches know that it is always best to be in cahoots with the forces of nature, rather than attempting to control them. After all, nature is much, much bigger than we are, and will always be more powerful.

Beauty comes from within, both literally and figuratively, and by working with the earthly and heavenly cycles we develop our skills at making the most of it. It may seem, at first, like simply too much effort, all this concocting. But it is time *very* well spent. When we are willing to make space for the moments—and, really, we are talking about small increments of time—to take our beauty and wellness into our own hands, we release ourselves from the tethers of misinformation and the confusion that comes with it. We know exactly what we are preparing, and why. One can never have too much knowledge, after all.

Once you get into the habit of crafting your beauty potions and rituals, you will find that routine has given way to immense pleasure—you will find yourself eagerly anticipating the cycles, getting excited in the planning, and fulfilled by the rituals themselves. There's nothing quite like casting a spell upon yourself! The very best times to conduct your Beauty Witch rituals are in alignment with the lunar powers that be. When blending brews, elixirs, and tonics, make them during the appropriate moon phase, as suggested in the recipes. When creating skin, body, and haircare, gather everything you will need ahead of time, and get ready to concoct at the new moon. (The exception to this will be potions used for clearing away energy. Those are best created during the waning moon, as directed.)

Allow new moon potions (with the exception of fresh masques and beverages) to sit overnight in a window, or outdoors if possible, absorbing the cosmic download of both the night sky, and the first light of dawn. Ideally, leave them in that spot until the full moon. This ensures maximum absorption of the cosmic lights, a full infusion of the crystals, and a rich marinating of ingredients. Working with fresh new energies, your potions are infused with vibrant life-force, building and gathering power as the moon grows. Collect your potions from their sacred spot at the full moon, and place them on your beauty altar. Anoint yourself with your new, super-charged allies. It feels gorgeous, doesn't it? And, I must say, you look *divine*.

# The Ritual Royale

Like throwing a saucy shindig, ritual requires a bit of planning. It begins with a certain preparation, rises to a crescendo, and ends with a blissful sense of contentment.

## Get Naked

Well, how else are you going to bathe? A good cleansing before magick is always smart, to clear away old energies and allow you to step into ritual renewed and balanced. Purifying herbs, such as rosemary, lavender, and lemon can be added either in a sachet, or as essential oils. Be sure to use an all-natural soap or body wash. And if you don't have a bath, a shower is just fine. Either way, focus on the water washing away any and all negativity. As you watch it disappear down the drain, ask for it to be rebirthed as healing waters. When you emerge, massage some pure oil onto your skin, adding essential oils if you wish. By the time you finish this book, you'll have a retinue of après-bath potions to choose from!

## Set the Stage

Gather all your ingredients, including base oils and crystals (if using), and place them together in something lovely. A basket, bowl, or a platter will work nicely. Bring it to the surface you will be using (your kitchen table works best), which you have prepared just beforehand with natural cleaners. For an extra charge, dab a drop of essential oil on it after it dries. Now is a great time to smoke cleanse the area, or energetically cleanse it with a lit sage or mugwort bundle (while you're at it, sage yourself too!) You can keep your work surface clear, or lay down a cloth that you will use specifically for potion making purposes. When choosing your altar cloth, bring in those charming colors and textures that you associate with allure. Make it superb, but be aware: you're about to make a gorgeous mess! Actually, altar cloths that are shaken or brushed clean, but stored as is will retain the energy of your workings, so don't be afraid to use a fine fabric that only gets hand washed or dry cleaned infrequently. As long as you adore it, use it!

## Light Your Fire

Have you already created your kitchen altar? Fantastic. Invite some friends from your beauty altar to join in the festivities—namely your candle, statue, and crystals—and nestle them in with the others to mingle. Add some fresh flowers. If you don't have them, culinary herbs, greens or fallen branches from outside, even a small potted plant will do the trick. Just bring some life to it! Now go ahead and strike that match. As you light your candles, feel the flames ignite your desires, the fire of creation burning bright.

## Focus Pocus

Now that your space is ready, take a very important moment to ground yourself. Whether sitting or standing, straighten your spine, drop your shoulders, close your eyes, and take a few deep, slow breaths. Ask the earth for her support. Simultaneously, feel both your feet and the base of your spine rooting into the ground. Visualize your roots stretching out to entwine with those from the trees outside, even if you are in a city. Now see them continue along, connecting to the root systems of the great forests. With each breath, feel the wisdom of the trees coming into your body. What do you wish for your potions? Keep it simple, keep it clear, and keep it positive. Get a strong image of what you wish in your mind, and hold it there. While you have the picture, now begin to really *feel* what it would be like to have it.

## Enchant Your New Friends

As you continue to see and feel your desired outcome, draw that collection of ingredients to you. Place your power hand—the one you write with—in the mix, gently touching each ingredient. You are attuning to the energy of the natural power inherent in them, and matching the vibration. Begin to speak your desires to them. The old literal translation of *enchant* means "to sing to," and has been used to suggest bewitching and spellbinding. As such, little phrases repeated will raise the power of your intention.

## Stir Your Cauldron

Now you are ready to concoct. Add your ingredients one at a time, keeping your intention focused. Each treasure you place in your cauldron brings its own special magick, so whispering its name and why you have called upon it as you create will elevate the potion's power. Depending on the potion, you will either be stirring by hand using ritual tools (p. 32–36), or swirling it all together in a bottle. Either way, mingle your ingredients in a clockwise direction, also known as *deosil*—"in the direction of the sun"—to bring the desired energy into the potion. Also highly effective for the clockwise motion is adding in a pattern that mimics the great cosmic spiral, and the ancient wisdom of the outer consciousness leading to the inner soul: the path leading from ego to enlightenment. Use the magick of numbers when stirring your beauty cauldron. Try 13 for its occult significance, 8 for eternity, 6 for beauty and harmony, and multiples of 3 for the Triple Goddess.

## Let It Fly

When the potion is well mixed, and intentions lapped up like water to tree roots, it's time to release it to the stars. If you can get outside, even better. This is the moment to bring it to celestial light, offering it up for divine infusion. With a high-vibration libation in hand, raise your glass to the heavens, and toast your celestial fabulousness!

## Tip Your Hat

As even the best *soirée* must eventually wind down, so must the beauty ritual. As you bid your esteemed guests farewell, you must always give sincere thanks. The sun, the moon, the planets, your deities, and your natural magick partners in crime have all gathered here for you, and have worn their very best for the occasion. Your graciousness will be returned. Be sure to ground your energy again when you are finished, and return everyone to your beauty altar. You're going to feel *amazing!*

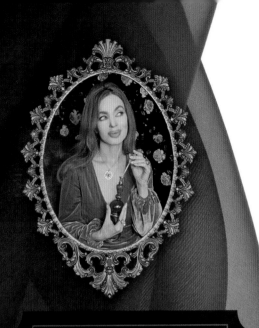

## Your Altar

Tell me, my Darlings, do you have a special place in your home for getting ready? What is it like? Is it a cluttered little area at the bathroom sink, overflowing with half-used bottles that you knock over in the haste of attempting to bound out the door? Or, is everything tucked away in a cabinet, hidden from sight, and, perhaps, a bit clinical? I'd like to invite you to look at your space differently.

Whether you are a pack rat or a minimalist, I'm going to bet that you haven't given much thought to your appointed beauty area, let alone the act of adorning yourself. Think about it: this is where you prepare to greet the day ahead, style yourself for an evening out, and where your bedtime ritual begins, easing you towards slumber. This is not your countertop. This is your *altar*, where beauty is invited in to be worshipped.

### BEAUTY WITCH SECRET

*Traditional witchcraft gives us the ritual of Drawing Down the Moon (and in some covens the Sun also) as a way of connecting to cosmic energies and entering a trance state. You can use a version of this to help prepare you for ritual potion making: Sit quietly, breathing slowly, as you visualize the full moon. See her coming toward you, slowly and with purpose, until at last she is positioned above your head, allowing you to receive the cosmic download.*

It's time to conjure your inner Cleopatra, and elevate your beauty rituals to a higher form of art, one that befits a goddess.

First, let's begin by creating your Beauty Witch altar. It must be functional, yes, but it must also reflect your desires. It should, above all, be beautiful. Your altar should be kept pristine with natural cleaners, always, and anointed with essential oils at the new moon. I particularly like cleaning wood and enamel surfaces with a spray of a diluted citrus and cinnamon blend, wiped clean, and then lightly touching the area with something alluring, along the lines of a sultry frankincense and rose blend. Don't forget to pay special attention to the mirror! Its job is to reflect your celestial beauty back to you, boosting your confidence, and returning your luminous gaze. Make sure to give it some love.

Next, begin to assemble your consorts. A statue of Aphrodite, Freya, Hathor, Branwen, or any beauty and love deity you feel connected to, deserves a place of honor on your altar. Have a small candle at her feet, perhaps in white to symbolize spirit, or a floral shade that you associate with allure. An offering of flowers, fresh or dried, makes a beautiful gift to her, and in turn, to you. Crystals are always a welcome addition to your altar space. Why not add a rose quartz to open your heart? A sunstone, to help your true, unique light shine brightly? Or a hematite, to keep negative thoughts far away?

And, oh, the potion bottles! Your delectable concoctions should be housed in only the *most* gorgeous vessels, like the fine perfumes of decades long past. Keep your eyes open for lovely vintage jars, apothecary glass, Egyptian vials … anything that appeals to you visually. Small trinkets that you love can be placed upon the altar also. Photos, cards, jewelry, hair decorations, and anything that appeals to your senses can be added as well. Just keep in mind the purpose of the altar, and what best illustrates your aspirations.

When you sit down, or stand in front of your beauty altar, take a moment to be present. Acknowledge that you have *arrived,* and that the ceremony of adornment is about to begin. Light the candle, and give thanks. You are here to worship at the altar of well-being, and unlock the innate radiance that is always inside of you. When you gaze in the mirror, you are seeing your innermost self, your spirit, reflected in the glass. Honor it. When you apply your potions, do so with purpose. After all, you have created them with magick, and that same love and intention should be present when using them. You have to carry the energy through from conception to application, and know that it remains with you as you journey through the hours of day and night.

The same ideas apply to your kitchen. I'm sure like many people, you've never considered your scullery to be a particularly glamorous space. And yet, this is where you will prepare beauty cocktails, brews, elixirs, facial serums, body oils, hair masques ... all of which will be absorbed by none other than you. Get the picture? An upgrade is in order. There is no need for a complete overhaul (though that may not be a bad idea) but rather a few carefully placed symbols of kitchen witchery. Using the same principles, bring the vibe from your Beauty Witch altar straight into your kitchen. Set up a little space to honor the charisma you are creating, the wellness you are embracing, the empowerment it bestows upon you, and all you choose to share it with.

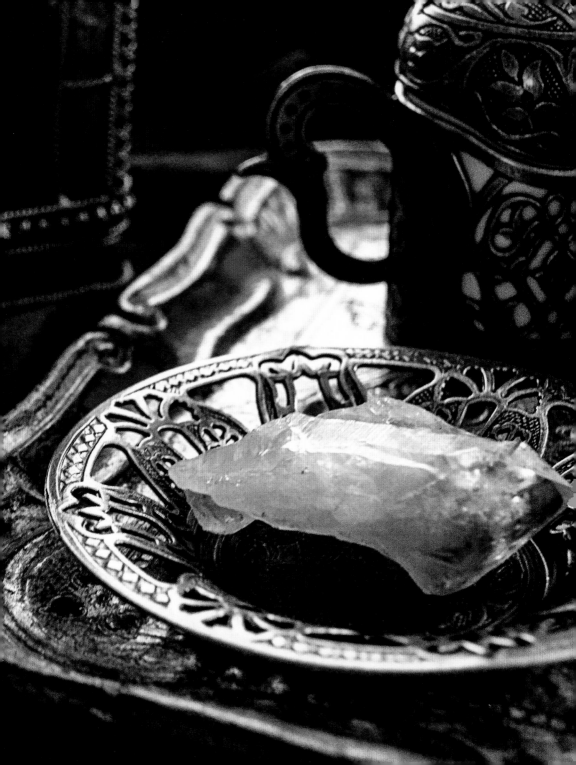

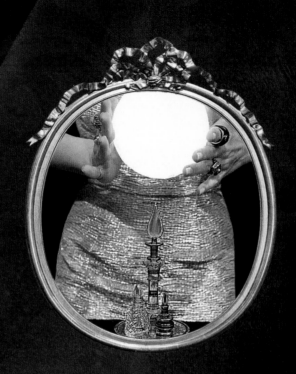

## Chapter Two

# The Moon

Oh, that white-hot light in the sky. That fickle seductress. Luna. She certainly has a hold on us. She draws us in with her provocative allure, then toys with our emotions like playthings. When we are filled with her silver light, anything goes: wild hearts, wild minds, wild actions. At first, she works subtly, slinking through the shadows. Then, growing, she steps ever more boldly out on to the stage, daring us to confront the obvious. She challenges us to face the spotlight.

She has been both revered as the mother goddess and reviled as the very essence of womanly wiles: a paradox of wise, maternal guiding light, all the while operating behind the scenes as a malevolent puppet master. So, *la lune*, friend or foe? Both, actually. It's all in how you choose to work with her, aligning your humble human self with her powerful

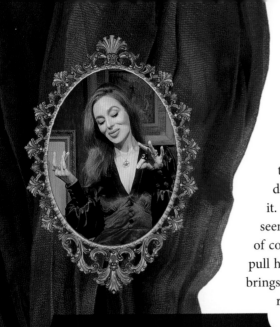

energies. She demands of us an awareness that too few possess. Above all, she commands respect.

The Silver Lady influences every living thing on this planet. Unlike the sun, she does not actually *give* light, but rather reflects it. Roughly 240,000 miles from Earth, she seems far away, yet is poised ever close in terms of cosmic bodies. This nearness means that her pull has a marked effect on us. Each lunar phase brings with it a unique set of challenges, and glorious possibilities for those who steer their ships wisely. With her 28-day rhythm, she aligns with the female reproductive cycle. Coincidence? Not a chance.

Though there are eight major lunar phases, it really breaks down into two halves: you're either growing or shedding, expanding or contracting, breathing in or breathing out, nourishing or eliminating. In terms of conjuring, you must ask yourself, *Am I bringing something toward me, or trying to keep something far away? Do I wish to acquire, or to remove? To attract, or to banish?* Your answer determines the most felicitous moon phase to work with.

# BEAUTY WITCH SECRET:

## MOON WATER

*Want to add a little cosmic kick to your potions? Set a glass jar of pure spring water outside the night before the full moon. In the morning, take it inside, after it has absorbed all the celestial light of the Moon, the stars, and the first rays of dawn. Use it wherever water is called for in your potions.*

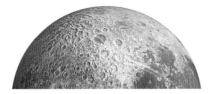

# Beauty Witchcraft by the Light of the Moon

## New Moon

*The Great Cosmic Tryst.*

Have you heard? A rather *steamy* affair is going on in the heavens. That's right. And it's been happening for absolutely eons.

Once every lunar cycle, the Silver Goddess meets the Golden God in the velvet darkness, unseen. These two celestial lovers live worlds apart, one ruling the day, the other ruling the night. All month long they journey to meet. At last, they are together, with only moments to share a clandestine embrace. This passionate, yet silent tryst will prove to be most fruitful. *La petite mort,* the "little death," has given way to rebirth, and the cycle continues.

It seems as if all the heavens are asleep. And yet, the first, tiny seedlings of what is to come have just been planted. The smallest particle of lucent glow alights the path for the Maiden Moon to appear, weaving threads of wishes into stunning bespoke couture for you to drape your heavenly body in beneath the brilliant stage light of the full moon. These are the very first moments of new life. The time to conceptualize what will be hatched at the full moon, that you will grow and nurture within the coming days and months. Though some immediate results can be seen, new moon spellcasting in any sign will fully come to fruition in six-month's time, when the full moon is alight in the same sign. The magickal child of this union poses the question, *what do you want to create?*

Oh, how I love this phase for concocting potions! It really is the ideal time to make a new batch and allow it to cure during the waxing phase, so it reaches maximum potency on the full moon. There is the energy present of working slowly, but steadily, towards a peak of power. Seeing results from any new beauty potion or ritual works exactly the same way: when you begin using or doing something new, you must give it time to fully work its magick and beget the intended results. The idea here is that you are creating something that will cure over time as it slowly, purposefully simmers. This phase also works equally well for trying a brand-new blend, or simply adding a new ingredient to an old favorite.

My Darlings, you have in front of you a completely blank canvas, just waiting for your masterpiece. But only you can pick up the brush and begin. And, like a great work of art, real changes take time. They must be given the space and the nurturing to allow their development. Consistent action on the physical plane is required to keep the momentum going, no matter what. Beauty ritual works the same way. When you start using a new potion or get into a new wellness groove you will immediately feel the changes on an energetic level, and will certainly see improvement, but the real results will appear in the coming seasons. If concocting isn't in the cards, then use this time to think about what you would like to draw in, and make a plan for gathering what you will need.

## When the Moon is New

PICTURE THE NEW YOU

FEEL YOURSELF LIVING IT

CONJURE A PLAN

SOURCE WHAT YOU NEED

CONCOCT POTIONS

Ask yourself what you would like to bring forth. What are you willing to grow? A whole new image? Fuller hair, clearer skin, stronger nails? More supple skin on your body? You decide. And begin to spin your starlit web.

## Waxing Moon

*Bring it to you, Kitten.*

Now is the time, celestial maidens, to implement the beginnings of a new you; one who radiates confidence, glows with starlight, and shines with vital life force, regardless of age. This phase is likened to Spring, with all her vivacious exuberance just waiting for you to bask in. It's the *foreplay*, my dear Witches. The gentle caresses that become heated, passionate trysts.

From now until the full moon, it's about absorption, nourishing, and drawing good things toward you. This energy forms slowly, gathering momentum as the moon grows. The Silver Lady gradually gains power, showing more and more of her face, and we follow suit. The stage lights are on, and as the curtain is slowly being withdrawn, the time draws ever-near for your moment in the spotlight. What did you visualize on the new moon? Whether it's a total overhaul, or just a few upgrades, use the first few days of the waxing moon to sketch it out in its entirety. Have the finished picture with you, burning brightly in your mind, as you take steps to attain it. Remember that thoughts without action won't accomplish anything! You will need to put in some effort in order to realize your dreams. The cosmos are on your side, though, and you'll find the mood around you is light, and quite upbeat, making it easier to get things done.

Over this next 14-day period everything starts to gather momentum, increase in strength, and grow to fullness. It's about expansion, so though it is a time of new beginnings, this is actually *not* a great time to begin a diet. Why? Because now we draw things towards us. This is a time of retention, not elimination. Rather, this would be the moment to *add in* a nourishing new elixir into rotation, start using a new beauty potion, and to embrace new wellness rituals. *Absorb.* We'll get to the shedding a bit later in the month.

This *is*, however, a fantastic time for growth. Your hair, your nails … every cell in your body needs feeding right now, so those little seeds you started can become luscious, healthy, full-grown plants. Practically speaking, it's about getting into a daily and weekly ritual, and sticking to it to see where it goes, ideally seeing initial results. Remember, you're *building* that glow.

Good news, *mes amies*! If you weren't able to concoct a potion or two on the new moon, you have fourteen gloriously advantageous days still to do so. Any time during this phase is still ideal for potions and beauty rituals that *feed,* so use this energy for potions that embrace your entire body with nutrients, moisture, and anti-aging properties. Your cells are able to absorb well now, so use the opportunity! I also love this time for potions that promote cellular turnover and growth. You will be attracting the magickal energies of each potion, as well, so keep that in mind. This time is auspicious for trying that something new to see how you like it. If it's not really revving your engine, then it can be passed on during the waning phase.

## When the Moon is Waxing

**Grow** your hair & nails
**Begin** using a new potion
**Add** in something new
**Start** a new ritual
**Build** your glow

## Full Moon

*Step into the spotlight!*

Mmm! Every Witch's favorite phase. Why? Because a full moon is full power. It is the height of potency for your beauty rituals, and a very strong time to concoct, particularly with your most precious and potent ingredients. The thing about the full moon is her immediacy. Traditionally, spells worked on the full moon are cast when rapid results are needed. It works the same way with beauty. And although beneficially speaking it is best to allow them to steep and release their potency over time, there is something to be said about a potion concocted and used on a full moon—it will indeed be super-charged vibrationally. This is why I love full moons for tending to the issue at hand, and getting the payoff fast, like banishing a breakout or treating a condition. Think in terms, too, of getting an exceptionally bright glow from a facial treatment, especially ample hair, and exuding star-powered radiance in greater doses. And don't forget that is a time of celebration, my Beauties, so when better to turn up the volume on glamour?

The full on, full power moon. It's time for your close-up. You have a glorious spell of high voltage potency right now, so use it well. The efforts for which you have so diligently labored are about to pay off. Though the night before the full moon is actually the most intense, you have a zenith of maximum occult power at your elegant fingertips for three full days, making it the prime time for a last-minute push to increase the effectiveness of what has already been set in motion, and to release it to the stars. It's the lunar orgasm. *Enjoy it.*

La Lune is at her most potent, and so are you. As she steps center stage, she holds space with regal presence, knowing that the spotlight is all hers. Your confidence is at its peak, too. Now it's time to pull out all the sensual stops. It is the summer of the lunar cycle, where we bask in the glow of our creations. Hair and facial masques, nail treatments, and body care goodies become stronger, more luxuriant. You're using your most precious, treasured ingredients right now, so think heady aromas, beautiful textures, and rare extracts. Swan about the stage, bedecked in all your finery, for now is the time to shine your brightest! The full moon, after all, is *quite* the extrovert.

Now bear in mind, the moon *does* control our emotions. This is fact. So along with the star power comes potential for tempers to flare, and with the unbridled passion comes the possibility of meltdowns. And, because our adult bodies are comprised of 50–65 percent water, and the brain itself is 75 percent water, the moon also has a very strong *pulling* effect on us. As such, the lunar force can also be quite draining if you aren't prepared. And even when you are, she can still knock you off your Louboutins. So, balance here is *key*. We need a bit of grounding in all of this. Unconsciously feeding the emotions with refined sugars, oils, saturated fats, and too many boozy cocktails (even magickal ones) only dull your glow, prematurely age you, trigger breakouts, and cloak your celestial beauty in lifelessness. Who needs that? Smart Witches opt instead for easily digested, nutrient-dense plant proteins, vitamins, minerals, beauty

## When the Moon is Full

**REAP** WHAT YOU'VE SOWN

**LUXURIATE** IN YOUR RICHEST POTIONS

**ADORN** YOURSELF IN FINERY

**FEED** YOUR BODY WISELY

**SHINE** BRIGHTLY

fats, and foods that stabilize you. The idea is to keep yourself strong and rooted, but never weighed down. Feed your beauty from the inside out, and you are feeding your power.

## Waning Moon

*The great celestial striptease.*

And, finally, it's time to shed some skin. You're coming down from the heated climax of the full moon, and a little catnap is looking *very* cozy right about now. But, before you lay your head down on that satin pillowcase, ask yourself: *What isn't working? What am I done with? What has exhausted itself?* This is the glorious, liberating peel, one layer at a time, until we are stripped down to rest in our divine stillness once again.

From now until the dark moon is the time for detoxifying, both on the surface, and—even more importantly—internally, as we prepare to pull our energy in. It is the autumn of the lunar cycle, and you are a great tree, drawing your energy away from your extremities and in towards the center, allowing the dead leaves to fall away. The show is over, and though we are still on a performance high, the stage gradually clears, the lights dim, and the audience heads home, having thoroughly enjoyed themselves.

You have about a week to continue to revel in the opulence of the full moon before things slow down. But be aware: you're coming down from an intense peak, so you *must* pace yourself. Just as we slowly gathered momentum uphill as the moon was waxing, now begins the slow and careful descent. Take it too fast, and you can stumble. Especially in pointy boots.

Take stock of what was harvested on the full moon. Not everything is meant to be a keeper. If you've given the pot time to simmer, and you aren't thrilled with the results, let it go. Embrace the cyclical rituals of shedding: use this optimum time to cut hair and nails, exfoliate *everywhere*, purify your skin, cleanse your liver and kidneys, and take salt baths, as they are all designed to release what is no longer needed. Even if you are enjoying cleansing and sloughing regularly, now you can really take it to another level—think fruit based peels and mud masques. As the voluptuous, fertile Mother slowly becomes the older, wiser Crone, there is less pressure all around, and emotions simmer down. You'll find it much easier now to take a breath, and see things clearly.

Overindulge during that robust full moon? Now, my Loves, is the very best time to let go of unwanted bloat, for the process of releasing now works in your favor. The cosmos will help you to eliminate toxins by clearing out your system, and, in turn, your skin. There is sufficient energy here which allows you to *let go*, be it weight, toxins, old skin, dead ends, and even potions and rituals that you find aren't quite working for you. It is also an excellent time to concoct potions which carry this intention, such as exfoliants, cleansers and detoxifying blends. As with the waxing phase, your clearing will gain momentum as the days get closer to the next phase, so it becomes even easier as you move along the cycle. Begin these cleansing practices now, and on the next new moon you can add in a magickal little beauty boost. Keep this going, month after month, and you will be well on your way to your most glowingly gorgeous self.

### When the Moon is Waning

**EXFOLIATE** FROM HEAD TO TOE

**CLEANSE** DEEPLY, GENTLY

**TOSS** WHATEVER ISN'T WORKING

**DETOXIFY** FROM THE INSIDE OUT

**TRIM** YOUR NAILS & CUT YOUR HAIR

## Dark Moon

*All is quiet.*

And now, for this one day, it is time to simply rest. As you prepare to embrace the new moon, everything must become very still, and as such is not an auspicious time for concocting. It is, however, an excellent time for getting rid of something once and for all. Focused intention, combined with the appropriate potion, can yield excellent results.

Recurring rash driving you mad? How about that sun spot which refuses to budge? That dreadful habit of sleeping with your makeup on? From beauty woes to kicking a bad habit, now is the time to bid it a final *adieu*.

It is the winter of the lunar cycle, cloaked in calm, hushed by darkness. What better time to burrow down, beneath layers of velvet and faux fur, for a much-needed rest? As you melt into dreams, your heavenly body is given the time it needs to rejuvenate from head to toe. When you awake, you are refreshed, revitalized, and ready for a new cycle. As the sage Crone Moon journeys beneath the surface, preparing for her rebirth, our stage is now dark and bare. A brand-new show will launch soon, but not before we take some time away.

In the three days leading to the dark moon, called the Balsamic phase, there is a very distinct winding down. These nights, dear Witches, are for staying *in*. Your party guests are now a good read and a restful brew. Your more introverted self can use a little hibernation at the moment, and will appreciate your consideration. Do you meditate? Fabulous. Go deeper during these days, perhaps extending the time you normally commit to it. Take thoughtful wanders out in nature, embracing her silent wisdom, and giving thanks for all the ways in which she has guided you.

## When the Moon is Dark

**CLEANSE** DEEPLY, EXTRACT

**SLOUGH** AWAY THE LAST OF THE DEAD SKIN

**SIP** CLEANSING BREWS, HEALING TONICS

**NIBBLE** VERY LIGHT FARE

**SLEEP** IN, SOUNDLY

Use this time for one last gratifying sloughing, eating very lightly (a juice fast would be *sublime* right now), and catching up on sleep. Give your digestive tract a rest. Schedule waxing if possible, as there will be less blood flow, and an ease of recuperation. Need a few extractions? They will bid farewell quite easily now. The extra cleansing clears the way for better absorption at the waxing moon, and the additional exfoliation here will allow for new cellular growth, all of which is integral to maintaining your celestial glow.

I love a good visual, don't you? As you are getting into the flow of the lunar phases, use this table as a savvy reminder of what works best when. Before you know it, you'll be naturally, effortlessly synced to the phases of the moon, and reaping the benefits.

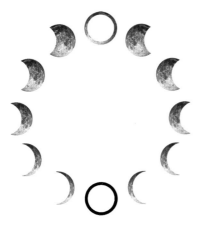

| WAXING | WANING |
|---|---|
| New to Full | Full to Dark |
| **NOURISH** HEAD TO TOE | **DETOXIFY** INSIDE AND OUT |
| **FEED** YOUR BEAUTY | **CLEANSE** SKIN DEEPLY |
| **GROW** HAIR AND NAILS | **CUT**, TRIM AND REMOVE |
| **STRENGTHEN** YOUR CELLS | **EXFOLIATE** EVERY INCH |
| **ADD** TO YOUR RETINUE | **MASSAGE** AWAY STRESS |
| **CONCOCT** POTIONS | **LET** GO OF BAD HABITS |
| **GATHER** INGREDIENTS | **RECYCLE** THE OLD |

# BEAUTY WITCH SECRET

*Smart Witches plan ahead. Gather a magickal assemblage of lunar-harmonized riches to have at your fingertips, offered in gorgeous treasure boxes or trays, and displayed for admiration. How about a Waxing Collection encased in gold, filled with nourishing body care, mixed dry facial masques (add the fresh ingredients just before use) and prepared teas? Its counterpart, the Waning Collection, sits in silver filled with detoxifying exfoliants, deep cleansers, and even a stylish retinue of trimming implements!*

As you learn to apply each of these lunar phases to your beauty rituals, the results are life-altering; both fulfilling on the inside, and *very* obvious on the outside. And, while you are making the effort to incorporate them into your earthly routines, understand that these phases *are always being applied to you.* Nature and physics will see to that.

Now, do be aware of one key factor: the moon will not always be in phase with what you are wishing for at a given moment. Planning ahead will get you far, but by its very nature magick is employed out of a current need. So, let's say it's a waxing moon and you've had a rough day. All you want to do is get that energy *off of you.* Can you take a detoxifying bath? Will it work? Of course it will. The practical magick of ingredients is ever-present; a well-crafted potion will always do its job. What you can shift somewhat is your intention. If this lousy day you wish to shed happens to be during a growing lunar phase, simply focus on creating the environment so that the good energy that is coming in *can reach you*—clearing a beauty block, if you will.

And there you have it, *mes amours!* Now let's make some Beauty Witch magick. I can promise you a *most* exciting series of adventures…

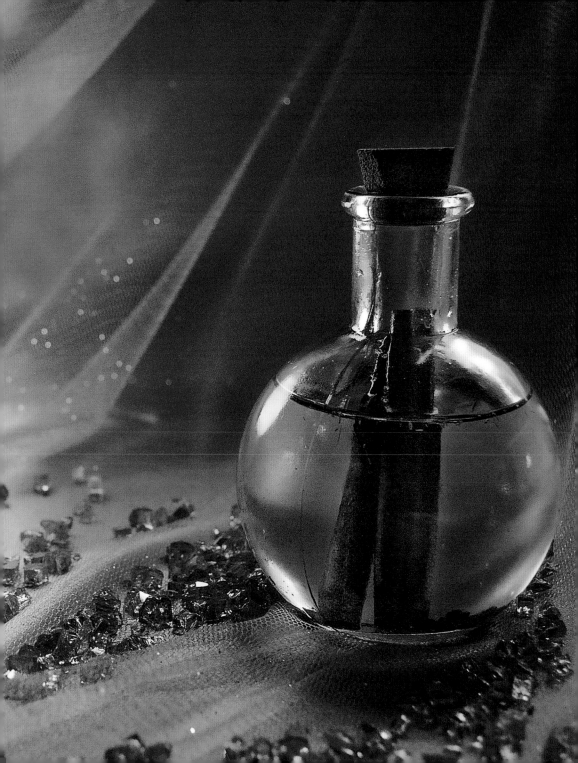

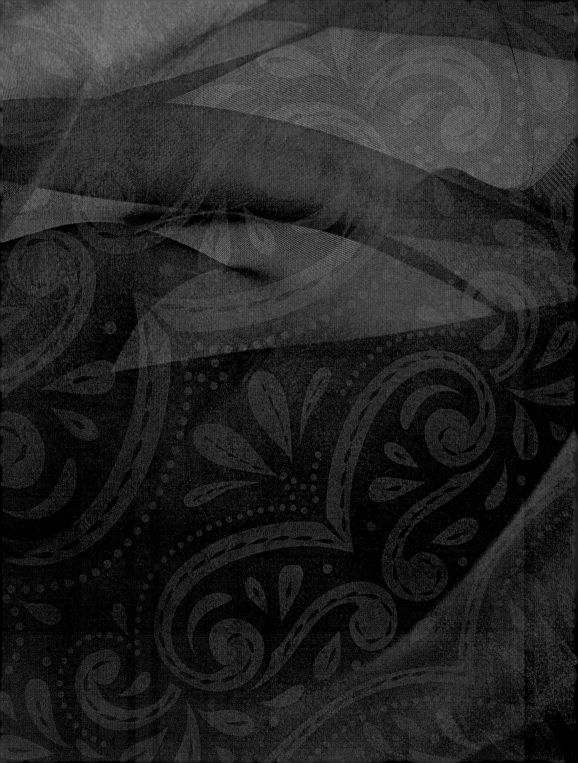

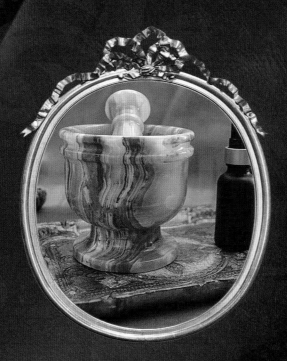

Chapter Three

# Tools of Divination

Like any great artist, a Witch needs the proper tools on hand to create the masterpiece. Because we are attuning to a higher energy, we must be specific. The types of vessels and implements we choose are almost as important as the precious bits we conjure with. Many of these little helpers already lurk about your Lair, but consider upgrades (see Resources p. 235). They are, after all, your magickal accomplices.

# Glass Bottles & Jars

When storing your beauty potions, steer clear of plastic if possible—for the planet, and for the integrity of both your ingredients and your conjuring. Glass is heavy, yes, and pricier, but it is natural, reusable, and recyclable. The higher vibration will harmonize with nature's gifts, and your investment will pay off. Colored glass is preferred for potions that marinate in the sunlight, because the darker tint protects the contents while allowing them to receive solar power. Clear glass is sublime for letting herbs and flowers remain visible, and makes for a gorgeous display on shelves kept out of direct sunlight.

# Labels

Even a seasoned Witch can sometimes pick up a jar of herbs with a quizzical look: "What *is* this?!" To avoid such awkward moments, I do suggest pretty labels. At least for the less obvious ones. Choose the colorful, simple variety, or the more ornate, vintage apothecary labels depending on your taste. Handwriting in a luscious ink is always a nice touch, as is adding magickal symbols. Just steer clear of generic white labels and scribbling. A neat layer of clear packing tape or decoupage sealant on top of the label will ensure a bit more longevity through washing, and for those potions that live in the shower.

# Bowls

———•◦▸◂◦•———

A close relative of the cauldron, bowls are the divine feminine basins from which abundance is created. Again, no plastic. Glass, ceramic, china, wood and clay all make suitably beautiful bowls to suit your style. This goes for pots and pans, too. Find those made of glass, ceramic, or my personal fave, clay cookware from the Mediterranean—the iconic Spanish olla is a stunning stovetop cauldron if ever there was one.

### The Cauldron

A symbol of abundance, fertility, and of womanly creation. In ancient times, it was believed that youth could be restored in a magick cauldron. We, of course, know this to be true.

# Funnels & Pipettes

———•◦▸◂◦•———

So, how to get those exquisite oils into a fetching potion bottle? With a selection of small-to-very-tiny funnels, preferably made from glass. There are wonderful long-stemmed ones out there. Less common are the petite funnels called pipettes, which are goddess-sent when transferring to travel vessels, and are well-suited to faeries, should you encounter any that wish to help you concoct.

## Mortar & Pestle

And now, the kitchen becomes erotic. The symbolic union of the female mortar with the male pestle further charges your potions with creation power. This classic Witches duo is a must-have for crushing herbs, seeds, resins, and the like into finer pieces—and even powders—to release their scents, activate their powers, and make them more blendable. They range in size and texture, from the rustic, stone Mexican styles that weigh a ton, to footed, ornate marble varieties. I like to have at least three around for different purposes. Get into the vibe when you're using them, especially for lusty love potions.

## Spice Grinder

Though I prefer a mortar and pestle for actual spice-grinding, these inexpensive little things work wonders for those moments when other methods don't quite yield the consistency you are looking for. I find them especially helpful when I need grains to be very fine for a facial masque, but don't have a large enough amount to use in my food processor. They are small enough to pop into a cabinet when not in use.

## Blender

Here's where I become even more of a stickler. *Not all blenders are created equal.* Most, in fact, do a wretched job of finely pureeing plants into a smooth liquid. This becomes particularly important when making elixirs. I only use a bullet-style vortex blender with a highly virile motor. Anything less, and you end up with an undrinkable disaster. For conjuring crèmes, however, I find an immersion blender to be the most compatible—not to mention the least messy.

## Spoons

The humble spoon takes on an entirely new persona when it becomes a tool for potion-making. Think of it as a wand, conducting energy into your potions as you stir clockwise to bring in the life force of the sun. Use simple wooden spoons for crafting your magick, and have many on hand. There are wonderful ones out there made by and for Witches that have magick symbols burned into them … go exploring.

## Spatulas

Like the stagehand that sweeps after the show is over, the spatula is as overlooked as it is integral. An absolutely necessary tool for not only coaxing potions out of a bowl, but for ensuring every last drop is included. Wooden ones are, of course the most charming and elevated energetically, but, honestly, don't work as well as the rubber variety. If you find you need a bendy one, try the somewhat-more-eco silicone spatulas. They last much longer than rubber, and don't leech as many chemicals.

# Knives

Your ritual knife, or athame, takes on a new form in the humble kitchen blade. Sharp ones only, please, for chopping, slicing vanilla pods, and cutting hard butters. If you were to find, say, a jewel-handled beauty to add to your magickal tool collection, I would consider it a justifiable expense.

# Hair Brushes & Combs

These mane-enhancing consorts actually have a history steeped in magick: practically speaking, they were employed by ancient peoples to remove excess oils as well as unwanted little beasties from the hair and scalp, but they also had another purpose; to pull negative vibes away from not only the tresses (which hold onto energy,) but also from the *mind*. Next time you give your hair and scalp a good brushing, notice how peaceful you feel afterward—it's no coincidence. Combs, of course, have developed over time into objects of decorative, ornamental accessories, often signifying wealth and status. The glamour associated with the hairbrush evolved more slowly, eventually to be used solely for styling, and therefore reserved for those who could afford hand-carved, bespoke brushes. Of course, now they can be found everywhere, lightweight, compact, and cruelty-free, but I do suggest an intricate vintage set to grace your Beauty Altar.

# Mirrors

———•◦►♦◄◦•———

Who's the fairest? Surely the magick mirror knows. The allure of the looking glass has been harnessed in divination, protection, and glamour magick for ages. Whether to foresee the future, ward off evil, or for admiring your own gorgeous visage, mirrors are essential to the Witch. A chic compact belongs in your bag, your car, your bedside table, and anywhere you require a touch-up glance that doubles as a scrying tool. It is important, as with all ritual objects, to keep them especially clean. Try anointing each of the four directions on your mirrors with tiny dabs of essential oils to best suit your purposes; my favorite blend is a bit of citrus for cleansing, followed by rose, amber, and frankincense for heightened beauty sorcery.

# Cotton Rounds

———•◦►♦◄◦•———

These petite discs are not the most environmentally-friendly, but, alas, they are quite necessary for cleansing and removing makeup, and rather useful for eye treatments. What's a smart Witch to do? Opt for the new, washable organic cotton and bamboo rounds. They often come with little mesh laundry bags (toss them in with the darks only) and can be re-used again and again, with the added bonus of being free of horrid chemicals.

# Spa Gloves and Socks

———•·◗▸◀◖·•———

Not the sexiest, I grant you, but I trust you will find a way to discreetly sport them when your hands and feet need serious moisture. Go for organic cotton or bamboo, and for the most effective results, lather your hands and feet in rich potions, put on the socks and gloves, and let them work their sorcery while you are sleeping. Alone.

# Facial Cloths

———•·◗▸◀◖·•———

Necessary for complete removal of facial treatments and masques, unassuming little face towels should be abundantly in attendance near your bathroom sink or washing bowl. Though bamboo, hemp, and organic cotton varieties are out there in droves, it can be a challenge to find them in sexy colors … sometimes you have to dig deeply. But snag them when you can, and buy extra. With regular cleaning in cold water they will last for years.

# Body Brush

———•·◗▸◀◖·•———

In addition to sensual body scrubs, using a natural bristle brush regularly does wonders for banishing toxins from the body and polishing the skin's surface, as well as increasing circulation, helping to keep unwelcome cellulite at bay. Sustainable, compostable, and vegan body brushes are widely available online and in specialty shops.

## Rolling Pin

What to do with that lovely old rolling pin your grandmother gave you? Heaven knows you've never used it to make a pie. I have a better way to put its magick to use: as a tool of banishment for unwanted lumpiness. Regular rolling on the backs of your thighs—or anywhere you need it—revs circulation and plumps the skin, reducing the appearance of cellulite. It works best just after a bath or shower and in combination with my potion specific to such workings, Temple Pillars (p. 138–139).

## Crystal Facial Roller

Like a petite version of a Crystal Visions facial (p. 89–90), a roller also imparts the high vibrations and beautifying benefits of magick stones to your skin, while using a technique similar to that of facial gua sha,

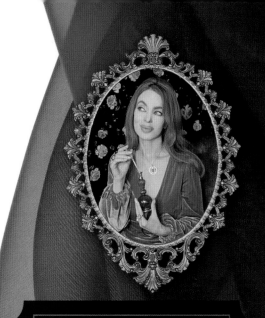

## BEAUTY WITCH SECRET

*During the dark to new moon, cleanse your ritual tools. Wood, glass, and ceramic tools can be renewed by first dredging them in Celtic salt, dousing them in fresh lemon juice, and rinsing with spring water. With other materials or when in doubt, a gentle sudsing in castile soap and a clean rinse will do. Cloth can be washed either in a machine with a natural detergent, or by hand (castile soap is lovely for this). If anything requires heavier scrubbing, use a mild castile soap, a natural sponge, and a good rinse. Pat dry with a clean towel, then let them sit beneath the night sky to receive its cleansing powers and be infused with the first rays of dawn.*

for a five-minute beauty ritual that instantly lifts, tones, and de-puffs. Choose your stones accordingly, and be sure to clean well after each use.

# High Frequency Wand

————•●▶◆◀●•————

Ah, *the* Magick Wand! Using gentle electrical currents, the high frequency wand is essential for maintaining your skin: with different glass tube attachments it detoxifies, treats acne, diminishes dark circles, stimulates scalp, decongests puffiness, firms, and stimulates collagen production. Ten minutes with this baby refreshes your complexion as if you just had a facial. Regular use produces cumulative beautifying effects *and* you can travel with it!

# Facial & Cosmetic Brushes

————•●▶◆◀●•————

I like to think of facial brushes as little magick wands with the ability to transform. Used to apply masques and treatments evenly, they are also genius for lifting away the thicker, outermost layer of a potion that has been sitting on your skin a while as it works. Cosmetic brushes are essential for spot applications of potions such as The Lion's Roar (p. 107) and glittery shimmer powders. Find cruelty-free ones with stunning handles, and display them on your Beauty Altar in an antique tray or a glided glass. For toting, keep them nestled inside a velvet, embroidered, or bejeweled pouch.

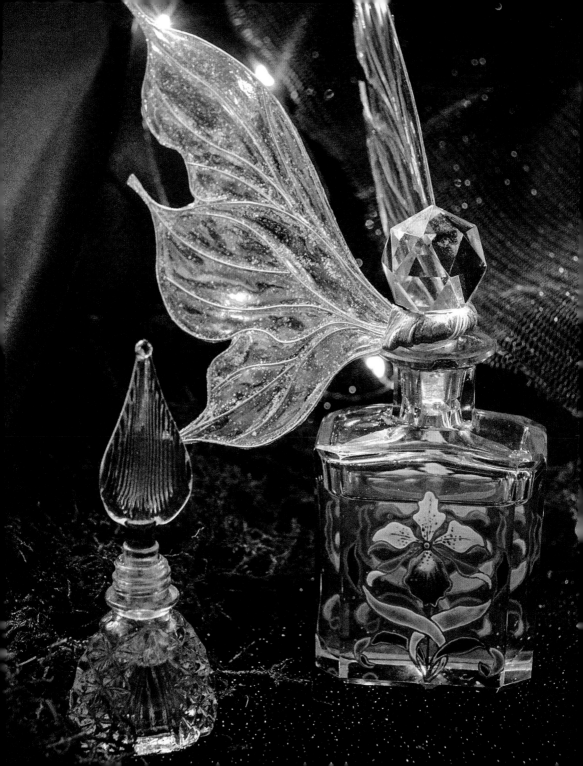

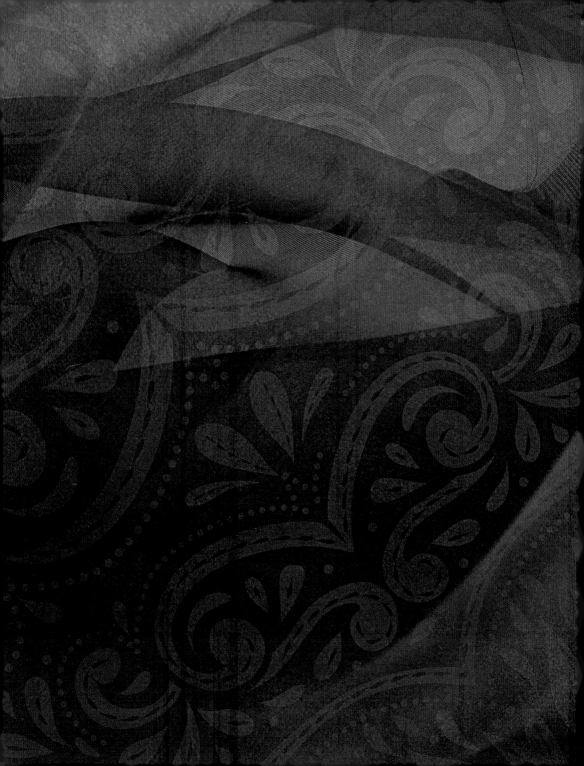

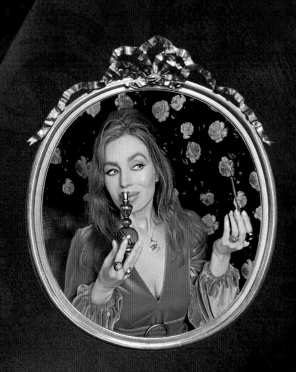

## Chapter Four

# The Potions

Now, this is where the magick happens. When plant power and focused intention embrace with celestial dance, bespoke beauty comes alive. Here, my Beauties, you have an immense opportunity to concoct pure treasure.

It all begins in nature's communication with vital life force from the earth, the sun, and the waters that bear the gifts of timeless beauty. It is at once effortless and dazzlingly complex. Plants carry information, but far too few humans are listening. By attuning to their wisdom, a higher level of beauty can be achieved. The results? Knockout.

Great respect must always be given to nature's gifts. She does not owe us anything, but rather, she will share with us if we harvest wisely. That heavenly, dizzying scent of a rose? The earthy, damp aroma of a tomato fresh from the garden? Those familiar, beloved scents are actually stress signals given off by the plant when a part of it is taken from the mother verdure. Bear this in mind when you engage in conversation with flora and herbage, and thank them generously for giving their light to you. Use their gifts with sage understanding, and it will be returned to you.

Potions must always be created with clear intention. It is crucial to approach potion making rituals from a balanced mental and emotional state. Remember: *the magick is only as potent as the magician.* Keeping yourself strong and healthy in mind, body, and spirit is key. You are sending energy directly into your creations, which will then go into *you.* You are what you absorb, so keep it positive. As you call in the assistance of nature, make sure you are up to *her* standards, or don't bother.

# Potion Prowess

Now, my Darlings, there are certain guidelines to follow to ensure bombshell potency in your potions, as well as a few suggestions for concocting that will guarantee success:

## Scents and Sensibility

Though the potions in these pages all weave the aromatherapeutic benefits of each ingredient into the blend and are created synergistically for their specific magickal and beautifying purposes, you can add an additional note of scent, if you like, to make the potion more pleasurable to you. Just be aware of what you are adding to the blend energetically by referencing the Ingredients index (p. 203), and choose thoughtfully.

## Bewitching Balance

In addition to being effective, potions should always strive to balance celestial energies as well as elemental forces. For instance, a blend heavy on fire energy can be made even more beneficial by adding a dash of earth to give the vibration a strong foundation, or a bit of water to guide all that drive with intuition, air to stir the intellect, and so on. I always like to punctuate a detoxifying potion with something that also adds nutrients, to keep a certain equilibrium. As you become more familiar with concocting, you can tap into your own rhythms to further personalize your potions. Each layer you add becomes another facet of the gemstone.

## Seasonal Shakeups

Potions for all kinds of beauty concerns are at your pretty fingertips here, though you will fall under the spell of certain ones that become your favorites—your retinue of consorts, beloved and treasured for daily and regular use. As seasons shift, though, you may find the need to mix things up a bit. Beauty oils are an absolute must that will carry you through all year long, but as the cold months approach, you may find that adding an extra layer to your skin by way of a crème is as welcome as a velvet wrap around your shoulders. Similarly, as the year heats up, your skin may demand a lighter touch. Vibrationally, certain potions will call to you at the right time—just listen.

# The How-To's of Hocus Pocus

Behold, the methods of magick for conjuring the *most* powerful beauty potions, every single time. Just be sure to always include three things:

**Make** and store your potions in glass or ceramic vessels, as plastic and metals conflict energetically with herbal magick and lessen the potion's efficacy.

**Cleanse** your magickal tools, during the waning-to-dark moon with only natural, chemical-free solutions, as detailed in the previous chapter. A rinse with spring water will clear your objects vibrationally.

**Follow** the Ritual Royale, and by all means, mes amours, enjoy yourself.

*Please note that all amounts in the Conjure section of each recipe are approximate.

## Beauty & Body Oils

Using a small funnel or pipette, begin with the base oils. If dried herbs or flowers are called for, sprinkle them in next, followed by any powders or resins. Then, incorporate any other liquids (such as aloe gel or vitamin E oil,) followed by dropping in each essential oil, one at a time. Give it a good swirl. For the finishing touch, adorn the potion with crystals. Cap tightly, and set it out to the stars. These steps become the basic template for all potion-making, with subtle changes in place for different consistencies. If you have included loose dry ingredients, you will want to strain those materials through cheese-cloth—make sure you wring out every precious drop—when the potion has reached full power, and before you begin using. Powders usually dissolve, but if they haven't fully, then strain as you would any other dry ingredient. As contents settle, give your oils a little swirl before each encounter to activate both scent and vibration.

**To use:** Apply facial oils directly to the skin, using about five drops. Lightly massage them into the face, neck, and décolleté in an upward motion. Then pat oils gently into skin, pressing rather than rubbing. Finish with a fluttering of your fingers all across your face, tapping lightly to create stimulation. Think of it as sprinkling faerie dust directly onto your face! Beauty oils take a little time to absorb, so allow them to work their magick while you tend to something else.

## Cleansers & Shampoos

Cleansing potions begin with a liquid base, such as floral or spring water. If using herbs or flowers, you will want to infuse them for at least 8 hours before straining. Add additional liquids (castile soap, aloe vera, etc.) and essential oils to the potion, and shake vigorously clockwise. If you are adding crystals or gemstones, drop them in last.

**To use:** The oils will settle, so always give these potions a shake before using. Pour a small amount into your palm, or directly onto skin, and massage with water to form a gentle lather, taking care not to dig your claws in—this can eliminate the protective barrier. Rinse well and follow with moisturizing potions. Witches cleansing potions are gentle enough to use every day, but do take care to not over-cleanse, which will only strip moisture and create a cycle of dryness.

## Masques

Always combine dry ingredients first. As you pour the liquids, or blend in mashed fresh fruits, stir with your power hand as you reach the desired consistency, adding a bit more liquid here and there as you see fit. Using the same rhythm as with beauty oils, you would then add other ingredients and blend as you go along, dousing with essential oils last and adding a crystal as the cherry on top. Fresh masques keep for three days at most, so depending on the need you can either use it three days in a row, reduce the amount of potion you concoct, or share it. I love sharing my potions with a few select partners in crime—a sexy little secret amongst confidantes. Dry masques, or dry masque bases, can be concocted in larger batches and stored in a cool dark place to be enhanced with live and liquid ingredients when the desire for it strikes you.

**To use:** For a facial or body masque, apply to a cleansed skin using your fingers or a brush. Gently massage into skin to activate their exfoliating powers, then allow the masque to set for 15–20 minutes while you relax. If needed, apply a second layer before letting it set. Dampen a cloth with warm water, and carefully remove masque, especially those that harden as they dry. Rinse well, and pat dry. For hair masques, apply to dry hair and scalp, gently massaging to ensure even distribution. Pile your hair on top of your head, or wrap it in a towel if you like, then let it sit for 10–20 minutes. Wash well with a mild shampoo. A light coat of your daily conditioner on the ends followed by a cool rinse makes a nice sealant! Towel dry, and style as you like. *Note: All masques should rinse fairly easily down your drain, but keep the strainer in to catch any strays with clogging potential.*

## Exfoliants

As with masques, begin by combining your dry ingredients first, then adding in liquids one at a time, and using the same methods of infusing your potion with intention. (If using a salt, waters or base oils, use lunar-infused versions whenever possible to increase potency—see individual sections for directions.) Exfoliants are designed to shed old skin and energy, but can also be used to attract by way of their ability to activate circulation, so adjust your intention according to the lunar phase. Exfoliants can also be made in large batches, providing they do not contain fresh produce or nut milks. Body scrubs can be also be used as bath soaks, and facial exfoliants can sit on the skin as a masque treatment.

**To use:** For the face, simply apply after cleansing with a brush or your fingers. Massage into the skin using tiny circular motions—don't forget those little spots around your nose, at the outer corners of your eyes, and along your jawline. Remove with a damp face cloth followed by a thorough rinse. For the body, apply and massage in a similar fashion, but then add a step: rake the exfoliant with your fingers in long, sweeping motions along your skin towards the heart. Rinse, but allow the oils to remain.

## Salts

The high-vibration of pure salts is made even more sparkly by a fave Beauty Witch pastime: bathing in the light of the full moon. Not sure if your salt is pure? If it is white as new-fallen snow, my Darlings, it's been chemically treated and must be avoided at all costs. Use only authentic Celtic, Himalayan, Smoked Alderwood, or Icelandic flake salts in your exalted potions and you will reap tremendous benefits (see Ingredients index p. 203). Pour your salt of choice into a glass or ceramic bowl and place it out beneath the full moon to absorb her potency. Though salt preparations are primarily detoxifying, I like to charge them during this phase to amplify the power, and to imbibe the salts with the immediacy of the full moon. Making a large batch of "moon salt," and storing it in a glass vessel makes it effortless to add an extra spark whenever a salt potion is desired. You would then follow the same flow of adding ingredients as above, but mixing either with your hands or a special magick "wand"—a spoon used solely for ritual concocting.

**To use:** Add a generous amount to a warm bath, then sink in and soak a while, allowing the salts to work their magick. If you are using a salt exfoliant, it doubles as a soak.

## Crèmes

I won't lie to you—crèmes are a production to concoct. They require a separate set of ritual tools all to themselves (as the oils can never quite be entirely removed,) make a spectacular mess, and spoil all too quickly. So, why bother? Because crèmes made at home using Beauty Witch methods—whether for the face, body, or hair—are *the* most powerful and effective you can cover your heavenly body with, the act of which becomes one of the best pleasures you can have without a lover present. Though some natural ingredients act as mild preservatives, without the presence of chemicals these lush concoctions have a short shelf life, so once again we can alter the recipe to make a smaller amount, or share the treasure. (Storing in the refrigerator helps, just don't forget about it in there.) To revel in the beauty of fresh crèmes, you will need two glass measuring cups or beakers, a large saucepan, a small whisk, a set of measuring spoons, and a bit of patience, as by nature, oils and water don't mix, so emulsifying to achieve the consistency you like can take some practice. But don't despair—it will be entirely worth your effort. Crème conjuring is divided into three phases.

**Phase One:** Combine the solid and liquid oils in one of the glass measuring cups. Place the cup inside the saucepan.

**Phase Two:** Pour the liquid (water, flower water, etc.) into the second measuring cup. Place the cup in the saucepan. Add enough water to the pan to cover the bottom third of the glass measuring cups. Heat both phases by warming them on the stove, taking care not to let them boil or become too hot. The idea is to melt the hard butters and wax, and bring both phases to the same temperature. Now they are ready to be blended. Turn off the stove, and transfer to the countertop. Pour the liquid into the oil, and whisk together to blend. Using your immersion blender, keep blending until the texture becomes creamier and thickens. It will continue to thicken as it cools.

**Phase Three** is the easy part: Add in essential oils, extracts, etc., and mix well by hand with your magick spoon. Fill small jars with your potion, leaving a bit of space at the top, and allow to cool completely. If adding crystals, clean them first, then drop them into the potion like the crowning glories they are. When crèmes are cooled, cap tightly and use for as long as they last. Because crèmes can spoil quickly (due to their highwater content) always use a clean spoon when removing directly from the jar.

**To Use:** *For the face:* Lightly dab onto your skin, after you have cleansed and applied mists, treatments, and oils. Press into skin rather than rub, and pay special attention to delicate areas. Follow with fluttering fingers as if you are sprinkling faerie dust (you are!)

to bring more circulation to the skin. *For the body:* Massage directly into clean skin, and allow it to absorb. *For hair conditioners:* Apply to the mid-section and ends only, massaging gently in. You can leave it on for a minute or two, depending on your hair texture, then rinse.

**Note:** Refrigerated crèmes will have the best texture if you use them at room temperature, but if you are in a hurry, any graininess will dissolve as soon as it absorbs into your skin.

## Balms

Beauty balms, much like healing salves, are made in much the same fashion as crèmes, with the notable addition of more plant-powered wax and the omission of water. Adding more wax changes the texture to one that is more solid, yet still soft enough to glide along your skin effortlessly as it drinks in the potion's riches. Following the same methods as above for crèmes, you will simply add the amount of wax listed in the recipe, and notice that there is no "Phase Two" (waters). From there, it is the same process of Ritual. If you are adding mica or glitter, it would be mixed in last, after essential oils and before crystals. Balms last for quite a spell, and do not need to be refrigerated. They can be stored in a larger ornamental glass jar—this works particularly well for body balms—or in several smaller jars, as you can use the same base balm and add essential oils to each jar specific to different needs and areas of the body. The recipes you find here conjure soft, sensuous balms, but you can adjust the hardness of the finished potions by adding a bit more wax if you like.

**To use:** Massage into skin anywhere, anytime you like.

## Sachets & Teas

Concocting bath sachets is sublimely simple. Unbleached muslin or cheesecloth cut into small squares are filled with herbs, flowers, and essential oils according to what you wish for. Use at least one teaspoon of each plant. They are then tied elegantly with a bit of natural string (hemp is a fabulous option) and tossed into a warm bath, infusing the water with their magick and heady aromas. They can be made in batches ahead of time, stored in a glass apothecary jar, and beautifully labeled for a quick pop into a bath when the mood strikes you. Teas can also be made ahead and stored, ready for use by making an infusion with water. You can do this one of two ways: by heating water just to the point of moderately hot (never boiling) then steeping the herbs for a minimum of 10 minutes, or by allowing them to steep in room temperature water for at least one hour. I prefer the latter method if you have the time, perhaps while you lacquer your nails and toes, or take little cat nap? (Your herbs will be marvelously strong, and so will you.) The potion is ready to be poured into your bath water once the herbs are steeped, strained, and essential oils are added. The same ideas apply for teas concocted to sip, though hot water obviously works best for hot teas and room-temperature water for those enjoyed iced.

**To use:** Float sachet in a warm bath, or tie it to your faucet as the water runs. The sachet can also be used as an exfoliating body sponge—how foxy is that?

## Mists & Beauty Waters

Born of mostly water, these potions are also practically effortless to conjure. Begin by pouring your base water into a glass bottle with a fine mist spray top. If you are using plant material or resins, place them in next. Add in any humectants or oils, then essential oils, and give the potion a good clockwise swirl. Drop in essential oils last, add crystals, and give it one final swirl. Place the potion out to the stars during the appropriate lunar cycle. Before each use, swirl the potion to activate the scent and vibration.

**To use:** Mist generously on your skin, your face, and all around you to clear *and* raise energy.

## Brews, Elixirs, Tonics & Cocktails

Witches Brews! Lovely high-vibration libations to be sipped for entry into a higher level of consciousness and vitality. Potions for ingesting are among the most powerful of all, because they work their beauty magick from the inside out. Conduct your ritual in the same fashion as with beauty potions, but now you are swapping your velvet boudoir witches hat for one of Kitchen Witchery—perhaps something in a draped chiffon, with a matching sheer apron to go with it? Brews and tonics, generally speaking, require some

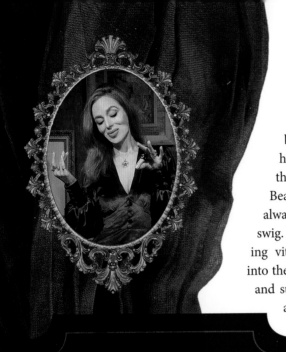

sort of steeping process, as they are usually built on an enchanted foundation of tea, whereas elixirs are often bewitched blender concoctions. Elixirs are created in high-speed blenders, in a similar fashion to that of the unfortunately-named "smoothie." Beauty Cocktails can be a bit of both, and always a magickal alternative to a low-vibe swig. They are each stellar vehicles for absorbing vital nutrients and healing plants quickly into the body, enhancing beauty with super foods and super herbs, and perhaps sneakily encouraging you to drink more water by way of a stylish drink. One thing to note, my Glamourous Ones: A Witches Brew must always, *always* be presented in a chic vessel. Under no circumstances should one be offered a magick sip from ... plastic.

GATHER ORGANIC INGREDIENTS

FOCUS YOUR INTENTION

CLEAR YOUR MIND

CONCOCT POTIONS WITH INTENT

ALWAYS SAY THANK YOU

## BEAUTY WITCH SECRET

*Add your most prized serums and mists to your masques for an extra infusion of power. You can even use one base ingredient, like avocado or besan flour, and add your serum and mist directly to it.*

# Oh, Honey!

The solar-powered nectar of our beloved bees is believed to be the oldest known sweetener on Earth, worshipped and adored by humans for centuries as offerings to the gods, potent natural medicine, and (surprise!) an elixir to ensure great sex. Considered divine, honey was also used to grant ageless beauty and youthful vigor, with an added gift of endowing one with a poetic tongue. Hmm. That may have added to its status as an aphrodisiac, yes?

Richly luxuriant and gorgeous, honey is sacred to Freya as the embodiment of the sun in the form of a golden sap; a "liquid amber." For ages, this celestial dew has been used to slay bacteria, heal wounds, cure sore throats, and treat digestive disorders. As a beauty potion, it works wonders to keep pores clear and control breakouts, and creates a beautiful antioxidant-rich glow that wards off the signs of aging.

What's not to love? Such a revered substance, unfortunately, comes with an ecological price. Commercial beekeeping can involve harming bees during the process of extraction. It is commonplace in such farms to remove the wings of the Queen so that she does not fly away. This alone is an unthinkable disrespect to Goddess energy.

Fortunately, there are beekeepers out there who are conscious; those who employ very careful and respectful harvesting methods, and have the awareness of ensuring not only bee's safety, but their nourishment and good health. But, as with all farming, these are not in the majority. Most honey you get off the shelf is extracted by whatever means necessary for the biggest, fastest dollar payoff. Making matters even worse, commercial honey is pasteurized. This high-heat process makes it (arguably) more attractive, but kills off vital nutrients, nullifying the benefits *and* the magick.

So, without piety—which I find a complete bore—I do omit the use of honey in my potions. This Witch awaits the day that its magick can be found everywhere, procured with only the highest regard for the sacred beings who create it.

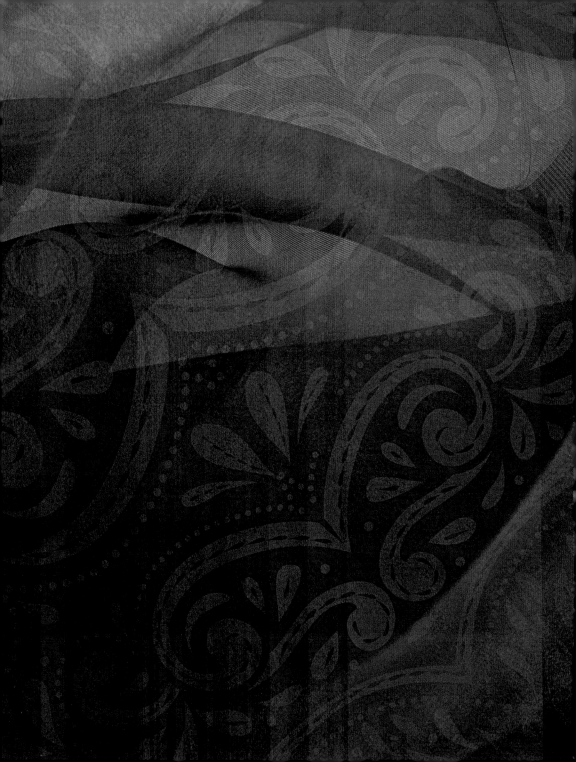

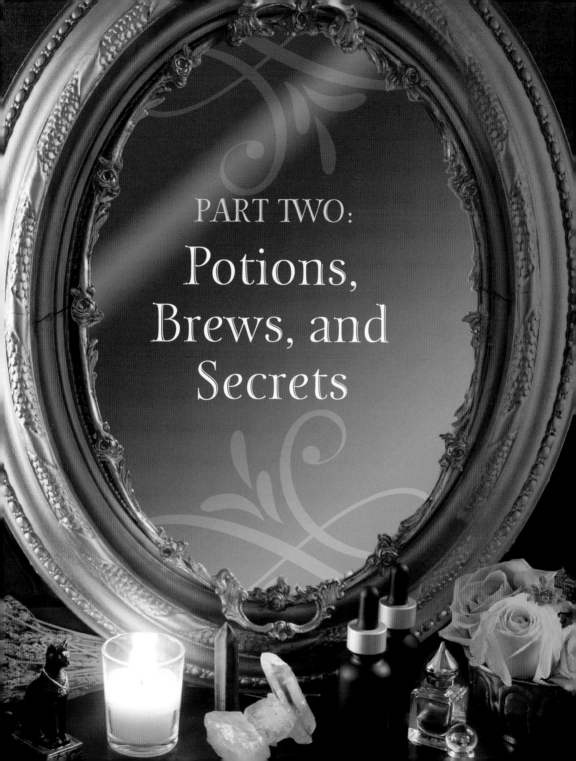

# PART TWO:
# Potions, Brews, and Secrets

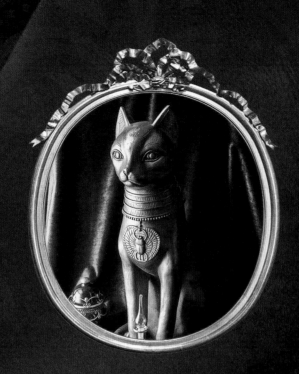

## Chapter Five

# Invocation of the Goddess

There would be no point in stirring a cauldron full of bewitching beauty secrets without honoring the great goddesses who embody that power: the ageless, timeless symbols that capture our admiration, those we emulate and call upon to bring us back to the true essence of who we are. It is, of course, no accident that love and beauty go hand in hand, and connecting with goddess energy reminds us of this. A practice of aligning with these legendary bombshells instills confidence and awareness of our own potential every single day, be it during joyous or trying times. And it's infinitely pleasurable.

I have focused on seven beauty goddesses here, though there are many. You must connect with those with whom you feel closest, the ones who appear. It may be just one very special Lady, or, during a lifetime, myriad co-conspirators—it makes no difference. These seven sorceresses have come to me over the course of decades, in dreams and in waking hours, whispering their secrets. They have lovingly, flirtatiously guided me to concoct my potions, with particular attention given to those in this chapter. It's interesting, and perhaps a bit curious, that from all over the globe seven have presented themselves to me: seven is a number of perfection, completeness, wisdom, and a cycle of renewal. I would encourage you, over time, to try each of these potions—of course you will have a favorite—as part of a new growth cycle for yourself; one in which you honor the goddess within.

When we hold ourselves in this light, by making beauty and wellness rituals part of our everyday lives, we harness goddess power, carrying ourselves with grace, dignity, and personal style, yet it is clear we are not to be pushed. Like a great jungle cat, it is best not to provoke us. All revered beauty goddesses have a dark side, and there is a way to use it wisely: rather than being on the constant defensive, this protective energy can be used to keep any potentially negative energies at bay.

To call your goddess in, or to honor she whom already guides you, create an altar space that she would love using the offerings I've included in each potion recipe. Invite her in with great respect, and she will be both your teacher and your confidante.

## The Triple Goddess of Beauty Oils

When it comes to divine beauty, facial oils reign as queen. Also called serums, they deliver their ingredients deeply into the layers of skin, and as such are considered the most potent in your skincare retinue.

These gorgeous potions are the High Priestesses of your beauty coven. There are three—representing the Triple Goddess—to be admired, respected, loved and called upon for their unique powers as the embodiment of the deity they are each named for.

Within these precious vials lives the most potent topical beautifiers known, combined for maximum efficacy and magick. Time tested and results-driven, they simply *work*.

You may find yourself drawn instinctively to one, but I would advise all three. Used in rotation, and aligned with their seasons of power, the Triple Goddess provides a sublime variety of natural magick to feed your skin as a whole, a living organism that is constantly changing. For instance, though I rotate my daily beauty oils in a manner one could almost deem religious, I find that I gravitate heavily towards Freya's Potion (this page) in winter, and Hathor's Potion (p. 61–63) in summer, as they are aligned with those seasons by way of the climate their ingredients are born into, and their energetic frequencies. All skin types will benefit from their magick, and it is never too early (or late) to experience such high-vibrational potions.

And, oh, are they sensual! Each is blessed with velvety texture and sublime scent, creating instant pleasure as you anoint your skin. This is true glamour at its finest. Just a few drops will do. Allow the space of several moments for your skin to devour them hungrily. Take a slow breath, lower your shoulders, and smile at your reflection in the mirror. Say thank you. You have just been blessed by the goddesses of beauty.

## Freya's Potion, Beauty Oil

The Norse goddess of love and beauty is one to get intimate with. A sexual powerhouse, she is there to fuel your inner fire with confidence, magnetism, and a good pinch of carnal know-how. Her potion is ripe with active ingredients that transform the skin, bringing the light of the aurora borealis straight to you.

**Season of Power** Autumn/Winter

**Offerings** Berries, sweet drinks, mirror, erotic poetry, chocolate, faux fur altar cloth, evergreen, amber, gold, roses, Fehu rune

Freya presided over the vast Northern lands, and continues to be a potent force in modern paganism. Fierce, powerful, and independent, this warrior goddess was the Queen of the Valkyries, who had first pick of the fallen, bringing the souls of the bravest dead to her great hall, Fólkvangr, in Asgard. These journeys with her shield-maidens through the heavens created the Northern Lights, as beams flickering from their armor lit the sky.

She rules sexuality and sex magick, though not marriage. It is said that she once briefly took a husband, and when he disappeared she wept tears of gold, which fell to the sea and turned it to amber. Her glorious chariot was pulled by two enormous cats, Bygul (bee-gold or honey), and Trjegul (tree-gold or amber) solidifying her place as the mistress of cats, and enabling her with the feline magick of trance healing. A sage who inspired all sacred poetry, Freya was also shamanistic, her falcon cloak allowing her to transform into a bird to fly between the worlds, returning with prophecies. As the goddess of prophecy, it is even whispered that sacred runes originally belonged to Freya, long before Odin obtained them.

Best of all, she's a firecracker: heaven help the great god of thunder, Thor, when he wakes her from her beauty sleep! But not to worry if you've missed a few winks: Freya's got you covered, literally, in a facial oil infused with flowers and berries she deems sacred, her celebrated amber, and the beauty magick of the great Nordic forests. (This potion is, however, particularly effective for use at night, when your skin naturally regenerates.)

Call upon Freya for heightened powers of sexual magnetism and prowess, mesmerizing feline energy, avian grace, and otherworldly transformational beauty.

### Ingredients

1 oz. rosehip oil

1 oz. meadowfoam seed oil

1 teaspoon raspberry seed oil

1 teaspoon pomegranate seed oil

1 teaspoon cloudberry seed oil

13 drops Nordic spruce oil

1 teaspoon vitamin E oil

1 teaspoon liquid pine bark extract

1 teaspoon liquid pine pollen extract

1 teaspoon vitamin C powder

¼ teaspoon amber resin, powdered

1 small emerald

1 small amber stone

**Intention** Renewal, collagen building, repair, protect, feed, age-delay

**Lunar Phase** Dark to new

**Conjures** 3–6 month supply

## Hathor's Potion, Beauty Oil

Ancient Egypt's goddess of beauty was really the Queen of Pleasure. She ruled music, dance, celebrations, sex, romance, cosmetics, perfumes, and the state of being, well, rather tipsy. Favoring red dresses and sporting a signature coiffure, Hathor ruled fun, plain and simple. But she was no lightweight: as protectress of women she oversaw childbirth, and as such embodied the Great Mother, her majestic solar disk headdress a womb to the sun, and a symbol of being at one with Ra. Her potion contains all the most powerful beautifying delights of the ancient world. Use it to heighten the sensuality of your day or evening; its intoxicating scent lingering on your exquisitely nourished face, neck, and décolleté.

**Season of Power** Summer

**Offerings** Turquoise, sapphire, gold, myrtle, music, dates, wine, copper, mirrors, red altar cloth, fabrics

Aptly titled "the Mistress of Life," Hathor had more festivals named in her honor (and more children named for her) than any other deity of the time. She reveled in her power as a woman, and knew that acknowledging her own beauty was not an expression of shallowness or vanity, but an outward manifestation of all her goodness within. Embody her quiet confidence as you gaze into the sacred implement of Hathor: the mirror.

As a sex goddess, she was able to harness the rejuvenating effects of carnal energy, known to drop her garment at the drop of a hat with a wink and a devilish grin, giggling all the way. She even once cheered up a depressed Ra by dancing and lifting her dress to flash him, causing him to break into a smile and stop his grumbling. The Mistress of Life, you see, never suffered depression or low spirits, and simply couldn't bear to see anyone else in distress.

Hathor represents the balance of opposites. Though a solar goddess, she also rules the evening sky. Along with her cohort Nut, she supports the Milky Way in the form of a celestial cow, creating a cosmic river between day and night, upon which both sun and moon travel.

On a more emotional note, despite being both a loving maternal goddess *and* the life of the party, Hathor has a shadow side: when she is angered, she takes the form of Sekhmet, the bloodthirsty lioness who punishes without hesitation. This speaks to the inner wild cat in all of us, and the destructive nature we possess deep below the surface.

Interestingly, her sacred attendants were both male and female, unlike those of any other Egyptian deity. Her priests and priestesses were artisans, musicians, and dancers of both sexes who brought joy to the people through their expression of creativity. Call upon Hathor to help you embrace your beauty and feminine wiles with love, finesse, and pleasure.

**Ingredients**

1 oz. rosehip seed oil

½ oz. meadowfoam oil

½ oz. avocado oil

1 teaspoon vitamin E oil

1 vanilla bean, seeds only

1 teaspoon hibiscus flowers, dried

13 drops frankincense essential oil

8 drops myrrh essential oil

8 drops sandalwood essential oil

8 drops rose attar

6 drops neroli essential oil

1 small, rough piece of sapphire

**Intention** Prevent and reduce wrinkles, firm, hydrate, protect, feed, cell turnover

**Lunar Phase** Waxing to full

**Conjures** 3–6 month supply

## Vanille Voluptueuse

The sublime aphrodesia of pure vanilla is one of earth's most sensual pleasures. Bearing the legend of impossible love transforming the divine into an orchid to provide pleasure and happiness to humans, this lusty flowering vine gifts us with slim, succulent pods that contain hidden riches: tiny black seeds filled with the power of what is known in Traditional Chinese Medicine (TCM) as "Jing", or the pure essence of life, believed to be found in black-colored foods. Release their intoxicating scent, as well as their beauty and love magick by first slicing the pod lengthwise, then carefully scraping the seeds into your potion.

## Branwen's Blend, Beauty Oil

The ravishing Welsh goddess of love and beauty did not have it easy. This is putting it mildly. But, through trying times and immense hardships, she chose to love. When we weather stress, it shows up rather immediately on our faces, and can stick around for the long haul if we aren't crafty. Add to that the visible signs of aging, and we really need to make some magick. Branwen is the embodiment of strength and resilience, and the symbol of death into rebirth. Her blend is powerful, yet laced with all the sweetness of earthly delights, and the renewal of Spring.

**Season of Power** Spring

**Offerings** Apple, rose, emerald, birch, fresh greens, spring flowers, white/sliver or green altar cloth, small cauldron, chalice, raven symbolism

Branwen followed her maiden heart into marriage in order to unite kingdoms and bring peace to the land, but it ultimately proved her undoing. As cultures clashed, this dazzling beauty was caught up in a battle of revenge, and unfairly blamed for the actions of another. She was imprisoned and suffered abuse, but managed with regal bearing to maintain her dignity and pride, all the while lovingly nursing an injured baby starling back to health. She whispered a message to the starling, who then carried her words to her brother, Bran the Blessed, of her situation. Immediately he set forth to rescue her, but his well-intentioned actions inadvertently caused a domino effect leading to great war, and devastation followed.

Though she was set free, she died of a broken heart. Branwen ultimately gave of herself for the greater good of her people, and thus reminds us to step outside ourselves to see the big picture. The careful, patient planning that brought her to freedom also guides us to keep taking action towards our own well-being. Call upon her to help you ease through life's challenges without wearing them on your face.

### Ingredients

½ oz. meadowfoam oil

½ oz. avocado oil

½ oz. sunflower seed oil

½ oz. sweet almond oil

13 drops carrot seed oil

13 drops pumpkin seed extract

8 drops helichrysum oil

8 drops carrot root extract

1 tablespoon apple extract powder

1 teaspoon vitamin C powder

3 small pieces of emerald

**Intention** Renewal, firming, reduce the signs of aging, hydrate, protect, feed

**Lunar Phase** New to waxing

**Conjures** 3–6 month supply

## The Goddess Treatment

As consorts to our precious beauty oils, enjoy these treatment potions that have been blessed by powerful goddess magick, whenever you desire.

## Lotus Flower, Facial Masque

Rising from the sea upon the sacred lotus flower, Lakshmi brings fortune, well-being, and enlightenment. Each autumn she is gloriously celebrated during the five-day festival of Diwali, peaking at the new moon, when thousands of candles and lanterns are lit to guide her path so that she may bestow prosperity upon all. Call upon Lakshmi by lighting her way to you, drawing her close with a beauty ritual crowned by this gorgeous Ayurvedic potion. She wants you to shine.

**Season of Power** Autumn

**Offerings** Sweet fruits (coconut, dates, figs,) candles, lotus symbolism, jasmine, richly colored fabrics (especially bright pinks and reds), gold pieces, flowers

**Ingredients**

1 teaspoon sandalwood powder

½ teaspoon ground turmeric

1 teaspoon coconut milk

8 drops jasmine essential oil

6 drops each lotus flower and root extract

1 piece clear quartz

**Intention** Brighten, age-delay, hydrate, new cell production, rejuvenate

**Lunar Phase** New

**Conjures** One treatment

## Moon Maiden, Facial Masque

The goddess Magu is the immortal protectress of beauty and vitality long revered throughout the Asian world. Known for her flawless face, luxe hair, and talon-like nails, she knows how to scratch your itch when it comes to restorative beauty. She planted a peach pit that grew into a massive tree, abundant with healing fruits which she gave freely to those who were hungry, earning her the reputation as the goddess of the elixir of life. Here's where it gets interesting: her name translates as "cannabis maid," for her use of the healing plant to cure sickness, banish demons, and provide spiritual enlightenment. One night with this potion will restore your skin to the state of total vivaciousness.

**Season of Power** Spring

**Offerings** Peach, deer symbolism, hemp, claw or talon symbolism, cherry blossom, porridge, green or pale pink altar cloth

**Ingredients**

1 teaspoon hempseed oil

½ fresh peach, or ½ teaspoon powder

½ teaspoon snow lotus mushroom powder

¼ teaspoon goji berry powder

¼ teaspoon schisandra berry powder

¼ teaspoon longan fruit powder

¼ teaspoon white peony root, ground

**Intention** Glow, revitalize, restore, anti-wrinkle, firm, nourish

**Lunar Phase** Waxing

**Conjures** One treatment

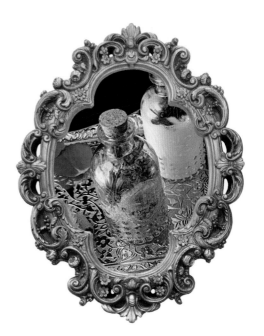

## Sweet Waters, Facial Masque

Oshun, African goddess of all things beautiful and erotic is a playful, flirtatious, coquette—and, lucky for us—quite accessible as "she who responds," so long as appropriate offerings and sincere compliments are bestowed upon her. She rules the "sweet waters" of rivers and streams, protects women, and is entirely irresistible to all who behold her. This alluring seductress does, however, get blue sometimes when she knows that the world is not as beautiful as it could be. Don't let her down! Adorn a gorgeous, glittering altar of gold and yellow, sing her praises, and for heaven's sake take care of yourself. This will make her happy. Letting yourself go will not please her, and who wants a great goddess of beauty to be annoyed with them?

**Season of Power** Summer

**Offerings** Sparkly things, gold, jewelry, gold or yellow altar cloth, pumpkin, sunflowers, amber

**Ingredients**

1 teaspoon coconut powder

1 teaspoon pumpkin powder, or purée (NOT pie filling)

1 teaspoon sunflower oil

¼ teaspoon cinnamon

juice of one thin wedge of lemon

1 piece amber

**Intention** Hydrate, firm, reduce and prevent wrinkles, polish, glow

**Lunar Phase** Waxing to full

**Conjures** One treatment

# Aphrodite Rising

◆•▶◦•◀•◆

Did you think even for a moment that the celebrated Goddess of Love and Beauty would be left out? Aphrodite chooses to drop in and share a few special potions for those moments when only her magick will do.

**Season of Power** Summer

**Offerings** Shells, pearl, rose, apple, pomegranate, myrtle, swan and dove symbolism, brightly toned altar cloth, jewels

Born of a union between sky and sea, Aphrodite made her debut as a grown woman, never a child. This ripe, lush female energy is associated with Litha, or Summer Solstice, and the voluptuous power of the full moon. She excited passion, and by this power ruled over all creation. Known also as the Goddess of Eternal Youth, she could grant beauty and charm to others. Swans drew her gem-encrusted chariot through the sky, creating quite a sight to behold. This one knows how to make an entrance, and can teach you. Aphrodite also likes mischief, and can ignite a little playfulness of the naughty variety.

A serious seductress and unabashed flirt, she took lovers whenever she pleased, delighting in the pleasures of both humans and gods. And why not? No one could resist her. If, by some strange reason (say, under the threat of death), someone could restrain himself from her charms, she simply used her magick girdle to bewitch them. Mind you, this was no "girdle" in the oppressive vintage undergarment sense of the word, but rather a ravishing belt made of precious metals and woven with the powers of desire. It draped suggestively over her graceful curves, mesmerizing the object of her desires. On occasion, she would lend it out to damsels in need, but only if she liked them, and they didn't arouse her formidable jealousy.

Now, of course, true beauty is always with us regardless of our adornments, though sometimes even the most magnetic femme needs a reminder. These potions, luxuriant and oh-so-effective, provide us with a ritual for those times when we need a little extra allure. Call upon Aphrodite to lend you her ultra-feminine magick, and she will be there.

## Irresistible Charms, Facial Masque

One sure fire way to conjure the ageless beauty of Aphrodite is hidden beneath the waters, in the richly hued world of sirens. Shades of emerald, sapphire and ruby entwine with beautifying minerals and plant proteins to offer you a visibly lifted look. Your face will glow like the moonlight across the crystalline surface of the rising tides. Who could possibly resist you?

### Ingredients
1 teaspoon kelp powder

1 teaspoon chlorella/spirulina powder blend

2 teaspoons cup meadowfoam seed oil

8 drops myrrh essential oil

6 drops rose attar or absolute

**Intention** Firming, anti-wrinkle, hydrate, moisturize, feed, protect

**Lunar Phase** Full

**Conjures** 1–2 treatments

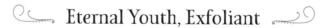

# Sea Spray, Facial Mist

Like a sweet ocean breeze kissing your face, this potion is a gorgeous pick-me-up, particularly during summer months. It will help to keep your skin gently cleansed while retaining its moisture, easing stress and nourishing with vital minerals. A spritz all over your bare flesh would be fun too, no?

### Ingredients

2 oz. rose water

1 teaspoon aloe vera extract

1 tablespoon magnesium flakes

1 teaspoon Celtic sea salt

6 drops rose attar

**Intention** Cleanse, hydrate, soothe, nourish, revive

**Lunar Phase** Full

**Conjures** 1–2 month supply

# Eternal Youth, Exfoliant

No need to bathe in asses' milk (nor the blood of maidens) when you have this bewitching potion at the ready. This everlasting youth soak smells positively intoxicating as it stimulates new cells, protects your beauty, and drenches the skin in sensual softness.

Though the exfoliant action sheds, the energy of this potion is full-on full moon, so don't be surprised when you feel your power rising. Or your libido.

**Ingredients**

1 cup Celtic salt, finely ground

2 tablespoons avocado oil

8 drops myrrh essential oil

8 drops cypress essential oil

6 drops rose absolute

**Intention** Boost circulation, fortify, moisturize, beautify, relaxing, aphrodisiac

**Lunar Phase** Full

**Conjures** 1–2 treatments

## Love Goddess, Hair Masque

When your tresses need transforming, it's time for a goddess-level ritual that leaves hair soft as the sea and cloaked in moonglow, the lingering scent of heaven seducing at will.

**Ingredients**

1–2 teaspoons (depending on hair length) coconut oil, warmed to liquid

½ avocado, very ripe and mashed

1 teaspoon rosehip oil

3 drops rose absolute

**Intention** Deep moisture, stimulates growth, shine, feed

**Lunar Phase** Full

**Conjures** One treatment

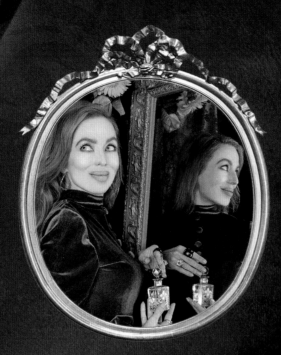

## Chapter Six

# Who's the Fairest?

The face is a great cosmic work of art. A unique sculpture, carefully crafted by the varied karmic dust of lifetimes, it arrives in this current incarnation entrusted to you alone for care. It is the opus of a master painter, lovingly conjured from the heart song of pure imagination, now on display to the world, revered and admired for its singular beauty. If you are seeing your face in any other light, my Darlings, you are doing it a great injustice. It is the face of the heavens, and must be treated as such. The shape and size of your features is irrelevant. What matters is how you present them.

Your facial veneer is a powerful reflection of your inner spirit. "Keep your face to the sun, the shadows will fall behind you," an oft-repeated quote by Walt Whitman, holds eternal truth. (No, Walt was not a Witch, nor a bombshell, but he certainly knew a thing or two about observing and conveying beauty.) I'm going to add to that: Hold your face up to the light of the cosmos, and you will always shine with starglow.

Is the value of this glorious visage merely that of a social masque? No, but by default it becomes its *raison d'être*. The face holds the singular distinction of being our calling card, our billboard—an ever-present advertisement for everything from our approachability and comeliness to showing off our intellectual prowess and singular creativity. Our every experience in this life is written upon it. The face belies our emotional state, how we see ourselves, and invites endless comparison. While we cannot control how others feel, we can take the reins within ourselves. The Witches power is to direct energy where we want it to go. *The face, in truth, can convey whatever we wish.* Make it a great movie screen upon which to project your confidence and well-being. Show the world how well you care for yourself, and you have now cast a spell to show others how you are to be treated.

Now, of course, in the privacy of our inner sanctum, we connect with our faces on a much more intimate level. It is perhaps the most intense relationship we have with our physical body—we inspect, fret, even criticize. *Was that line there yesterday? Where did that blemish come from?* We always want to look our absolute best; anyone who tells you differently is fibbing at the level of a politician. I will encourage you to sit at your beauty altar each morning and take a good look at what your countenance is telling you. Let me guess: it needs more sleep, more water, less stress? These are all so common its actually almost funny. Almost. Except that life is continually happening. So, no despair, no ignoring. Instead, don your conical hat and give your face what it asks for. No one else can do it. And, like all ever-growing life forms, its needs will change often, keeping you perpetually on your toes. The beauty of it, really, is that it forces us once again to take our wellness into our own hands, a reminder that we *can* control to a great extent how we appear. Lavish your favorite features, elevate your skincare to that of religious practice, embrace what makes you interesting, and by all means, if something truly makes you miserable, change it. Let go of the absurd notion that as we get older our beauty somehow diminishes, or worse, disappears entirely. *Our beauty evolves.* The whole idea of anti-aging cannot be taken literally, because there is no such thing. Rather it must be translated, wisely, as the unwillingness to age anything less than amazingly, embracing youth not just where the world can see it but on the inside, where it truly resides. That balance between experienced, worldly wisdom and youthful enthusiasm is knock-their-socks-off sexy. *Le femme d'un certain âge* has it. But only if she takes stellar care of herself. Starting now.

# The Ritual of the Face

From the tips of your tootsies to the base of your crowning glory, skin craves moisture. It lives on it. If you've never given it much thought, consider this: dehydration causes premature aging. And your skin begins the aging process as early as your late 20's.

If you have dry or aging skin, you know all about this, for you are likely in a constant act of trying to give your skin the emollients it needs. Oily and eruptive skin needs it too—depriving it of essential moisture only causes it to over-dry, which then tells the skin to create more oil, creating a vicious cycle.

Of course, we must be hydrated internally for it all to work most effectively, but what you put on your skin is also crucial. Harsh chemicals, alcohol, and synthetics can deplete your skin of what it craves most. Fortunately, the opposite is even more powerful: rich fats, humectants, and nutrient-dense natural moisturizers will keep your skin soft and supple, prevent breakouts, stave off and even repair those fine lines that become more pronounced when the skin is thirsty. A twice-daily ritual is a Witch's best ally for keeping skin at its best, with a few little spellbound spa treatments here and there for heightened beauty rapture:

## Cleanse

A good cleansing is an essential foundation for your facial rituals, however, it varies by skin type, season, and personal preference. While those who possess very dry skin benefit from just a splash of warm water, most need a bit of gentle cleansing, particularly if you wear makeup. From extremely light micellar water to a heavier oil cleanse, there is a potion in the following recipes to suit your every need. I personally use Eau de Vie (p. 80) twice daily all year around, adding in Cleansing Nectar (p. 80–81) when the weather begins to get cold and dry, and on occasion Facial Bath (p. 81) if I find my skin requires a bit more cleansing, such as after heavy exercise or a very hot, sticky day.

## Mist

Toning mists are so often forgotten, by way of presuming they are unnecessary. *Au contraire!* They are actually an integral part of the ritual. And you wouldn't bypass a step in your magick, now would you? Facial mists that are created with nourishing ingredients actually add a layer of nutrition and hydration, effectively restoring the pH level to your skin after cleansing. But it gets better: the act of dampening the skin just before applying beauty oils makes them penetrate deeper—as much as ten times—making those precious concoctions *even more* powerful. The cherry on top? A spritz here and there throughout your day will revive your face and your spirit. Make it a habit to never skip this stage in your beauty ritual, and your skin will reward you.

## Treat

Occasionally, even the most bewitching complexion encounters a foe. Appearing in the form of a blemish, irritation, or stubborn dry patch, these areas must be tended to immediately, taking care not to focus angry energy on your face. Spot-treating with essential and nutrient-dense oils will help to heal these *petites blessures* quickly and with aplomb.

## Infuse

Here is where the serious magick comes in: specialty beauty oils (or serums) that work hard on your behalf, delivering the most intense natural remedies for repair and prevention possible. Combined for sublime efficacy, they work deeply to penetrate your skin with supreme nutrition for cumulative results. They also work beautifully as pick-me ups whenever your skin needs reviving, adding a touch of spellbinding glow just when you need it. Much like diet, skin requires complete nutrition, so by rotating your beauty oils you gift it with a wide variety of support for keeping it healthy and gorgeous. They truly are the Witches secret to otherworldly radiance!

## Protect

As your beauty oils are the stars that perform and delight with highly skilled expertise, you then need a protector at the stage door—a bouncer, if you will. Crèmes act as guards for your skin, keeping damaging UV rays and environmental stressors at bay while ensuring that moisture stays intact. Even for oily skin, a dab of crème is a must for these reasons. One with natural sunscreen, a pure humectant, generous doses of antioxidants, and a lipid that acts as an occlusive—a moisture barrier to keep skin from losing hydration—will work hard to protect your beauty. Hold them in high regard, and be sure to tip generously.

## Remove

When you wish to unwind, a gentle but seriously *thorough* makeup remover is needed. One that requires no friction to your delicate eye area whatsoever, but instead melts away debris easily and leaves behind a light layer of emollients is a wise and sensual choice. And, my Loves, never, ever, skip this step! Forget the notion of slept-in makeup somehow being cool. It's not. It will only accelerate lines and slack skin and cause next-morning puffiness, which will then leave you in a panic to somehow undo. And frantic behavior is decidedly uncool. A Smart Witch takes exquisite care of her face, always.

## Spellbound Spa

Once weekly, at the very least, your Beauty Altar should host a very special *soirée*: the home spa. This is the time for paying extra attention to your beauty needs (and desires) with relaxing treatments for your entire body. If you aren't already taking time out for these rituals, you simply must, beginning this week. Chose a time you can set aside peacefully, and luxuriate in glamourous concoctions. My personal favorite is to employ a delicious facial exfoliant followed by a masque and let it set while luxuriating in a potion-filled bath.

Whoever said bombshells were impractical was dead wrong—this is a masterful use of time, no?

## Salon de Beauté

Then, of course, there are the occasional wanderings outside the Lair, seeking beauty care in intriguing new ways. The red carpet leads directly to the house of worship best known by its common name: The Spa. But only the best will do for a Witch; choose a holistic, organic spa that uses natural products and healing techniques. There are so many cropping up these days, and not just in major cities. Look for facials that incorporate plant-based potions with microcurrent, fruit acid peels, gua sha, facial massage, cosmetic acupuncture, microdermabrasion, crystals, and energy work. A reputable spa will offer a consultation with their practitioners to determine the best choices for you. And use your intuition. If someone is pushing for anything other than the gentlest version of a first-time treatment, or is shoving high-priced products at you bid them *adieu*. You can smell someone out for the upsell a mile away. And you can concoct *much* better potions.

# To Banish a Blemish

Nasty spot about to make an appearance on your gleaming face? No, no. This will never do. Nip it in the bud with this highly reliable Beauty Witch spell; complete with a potion and a magick wand.

- Clean the area thoroughly with Facial Bath (p. 81). Rinse well.

- Apply a dab of the following Banish Blemish potion:

  ½ teaspoon Moroccan red clay

  ½ teaspoon water

  3 drops lavender essential oil

- Let the potion sit until dried, approximately three minutes, while closing your eyes and repeating this chant:

  *Out, out damned spot!*

  *Be gone at once*

  *I'll miss you not*

Must you say the words? No, but they carry power. And it's fun. You can chant silently if you like.

- Soak a face towel in warm water, and wring it out. Press the warm towel onto the clay-covered area to soften. Gently remove all the clay, and rinse well. Lightly pat dry.

- Use a high frequency wand (pink tube) directly on the blemish for 60 seconds.

- Treat the spot with lavender essential oil.

* *For deep or large blemishes, it may be necessary to repeat this ritual for a period of days. To speed the process, leave the potion on for hours at a time, or overnight. Just be very careful to soften the clay thoroughly before attempting to remove.*

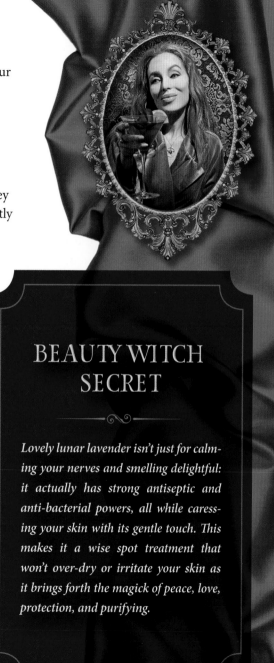

## BEAUTY WITCH SECRET

*Lovely lunar lavender isn't just for calming your nerves and smelling delightful: it actually has strong antiseptic and anti-bacterial powers, all while caressing your skin with its gentle touch. This makes it a wise spot treatment that won't over-dry or irritate your skin as it brings forth the magick of peace, love, protection, and purifying.*

# Eau de Vie, Facial Water

Behold the gentlest cleansing your skin can ask for—the classic French micellar water. The Witches version is, of course, sans chemicals and fillers and instead infused with magick. This lovely, light potion bathes your skin in hydration without oiliness and works wonders on all skin, never stripping away essential moisture while removing all traces of makeup and mire.

**Ingredients**

2 oz. rosewater

2 teaspoons aloe vera extract

1 teaspoon vegetable glycerin

½ teaspoon cold-pressed extra virgin olive oil

**Intention** Gently cleanse, hydrate, protect

**Lunar Phase** Waning

**Conjures** 1 month supply

# Cleansing Nectar, Cleansing Oil

What a sensual, glorious way to awaken your beauty! A gently stimulating massage twice daily with this potion will give you a fresh canvas as it softly cleanses, encourages cellular turnover, feeds your skin, and whispers away stress. You can remove it with a warm, damp, cloth or a swipe of a rosewater-kissed facial pad. It is suitable for all skin types, particularly during cold, dry months. And it feels like heaven.

**Ingredients**

2½ oz. grapeseed oil

1 oz. castor oil

20 drops lavender oil

**Intention** gently cleanse, unclog pores, stimulate circulation, balance moisture levels

**Lunar Phase** Waning

**Conjures** 1–2 month supply

## Bain du Visage, Cleansing Wash

For those days when you appreciate a sudsier kind of clean, use this light-as-air potion to bathe your pores a bit more deeply while keeping moisture levels right where they should be, even for oily skin. Squeaky clean? Well, no. That would be more for … windows.

### Ingredients

1½ oz. rosewater

.05 oz. aloe vera liquid extract

.05 oz. pure castile soap

8 drops lavender oil

8 drops chamomile oil

**Intention** purify, soothe, balance moisture levels

**Lunar Phase** Waning

**Conjures** 1–2 month supply

## Bewitching Beauty Mist, Toning Mist

Toss your head back in sheer joy and let this stunning potion kiss you! Lusciously scented and ever-so-soft, a superior blend of beautifiers conspire to veil your face and neck in a swathe of nutritious moisture. A quick spritz lays the foundation for your beauty oils and makes for a delightful pick-me-up whenever you wish, so be sure to keep it close for a reviving glow whenever the mood strikes you.

**Ingredients**

2 oz. rosewater

1 teaspoon vegetable glycerin

½ teaspoon avocado oil

8 drops neroli essential oil

8 drops helichrysum essential oil

8 drops blue tansy essential oil

6 drops ginseng extract

1 small piece each of ruby, sapphire, and emerald

**Intention** Refresh, revive, glow, moisturize, balance, soothe, hydrate, de-stress

**Lunar Phase** New

**Conjures** 1–2 month supply

## Crème de la Sorcière, Face Crème

Like the purrfect coat for every ensemble, this luxe potion protects with sorceress style: a potent outer layer to lock in the beauty magick of what's underneath, from the delicate lingerie of your beauty mist to the couture of this season's beauty oils. Intensely moisturizing without clogging pores, this layer feeds skin continuously with the cumulative powers of plant magick from around the globe. Think of it as the only cloak you need for any occasion.

**Ingredients**

**Phase One**

⅓ cup cacao butter

1 tablespoon candelilla wax

½ cup grapeseed oil

¼ cup avocado oil

**Phase Two**

⅔ cup rosewater

⅓ cup aloe vera gel

**Phase Three**

1 teaspoon ginseng extract

1 teaspoon hyaluronic acid

20 drops ylang ylang essential oil

20 drops carrot seed essential oil

**Intention** Intense hydration, moisture seal, mild sun protection, firming, plumping

**Lunar Phase** Full

**Conjures** 6 month supply

## Strip Tease, Eye Makeup Remover

When it's time for the slow peel, take it all off with élan—the soft tease that leads to sheer nakedness. This third-eye opener blend of nourishing oils is a simply delicious way to remove every last trace of eye makeup (including lash glue!) while coaxing alluring growth to your fluttering feathers. With regular use, it even fills in sparse brows. And you know how devastatingly sexy an abundant arch can be.

**Ingredients**

2 oz. coconut oil, solid

13 drops lavender oil

8 drops jasmine absolute

**Intention** Gently dissolve makeup and remove irritants, moisturize, grow lashes & brows

**Lunar Phase** New

**Conjures** 1–2 month supply

## Ambrosia Amour, Facial Masque

Joyous as a tumble in the tall grass on a warm afternoon, this potion is a rite of pure pleasure—and, like a secret tryst, it has an incredible effect on your skin. Use this to balance and brighten with age-fighting superpowers, suitable for all skin types. Was that you I saw in the meadow?

### Ingredients

1 teaspoon fresh peach, very ripe, or 1 teaspoon peach powder

1 teaspoon banana, very ripe, or 1 teaspoon banana powder

1 tablespoon unsweetened almond milk

3 drops lemon essential oil

6 drops neroli essential oil

**Intention** Clear pores, cellular turnover, moisturize, glow

**Lunar Cycle** New to full

**Conjures** 1 treatment

# That Old Black Magick,
## ᏅᎾ Facial Masque & Exfoliant ᎾᏴ

In the deep dark of the detox cycle, your skin needs a major dose of mystical mojo. Regardless of skin type, a good cleansing must be performed, at just the right time, to clear away old energies, whatever form they take. This delicately scented potion does just that, leaving your skin polished and poreless, ready for the next phase to begin.

### Ingredients

1 teaspoon activated charcoal, or two opened capsules

½ teaspoon Moroccan red clay

½ teaspoon aloe vera extract

½ teaspoon grapeseed oil

8 drops lavender essential oil

**Intention** Deep cleanse, detoxify, exfoliate

**Lunar Phase** Dark

**Conjures** 1–2 treatments

# Calm In The Storm,
## ᏅᎾ Facial Masque & Exfoliant ᎾᏴ

Some days tax the reserves of even the most resilient Witch, and have the unenviable side effect of upsetting her complexion. This, of course, is unacceptable. Banish stress from your day, and your face, with this soothing masque while soaking in a calming bath—you will emerge with a calmed, detoxified, and lifted visage, with your entire heavenly body restored. Add a beauty cocktail to the ritual for even more sublime stress relief.

**Ingredients**

¼ cup rolled oats, ground, or oat flour

¼ cup garbanzo flour

1 teaspoon French green clay

6 drops lavender essential oil

¼ cup spring water, or as desired

**Intention** Purify, tighten, calm

**Lunar Phase** Waning

**Conjures** 2 treatments

## Solar Sorcery, Facial Masque

When a Witch does a striptease, it is truly something to behold. A ritual masque for shedding old skin couldn't come in a sexier potion: a voluptuous blend of seductive fruits acts as a natural, high-vibrational peel which also provides a protective moisture barrier, lighting the path to renewed vibrance.

**Ingredients**

½ cup pineapple, or 1 teaspoon pineapple powder

½ cup mango, or 1 teaspoon mango powder

1 teaspoon white clay

½ teaspoon sunflower oil

*Note: If using fruit powders, increase the oil to 3 teaspoons*

**Intention** Exfoliation, firming, cell renewal, moisture

**Lunar Phase** Waning

**Conjures** 1 treatment

## ᕙ Blue Moon, Facial Masque ᕗ

Whoever said caring for oily skin had to be an antiseptic chore? Banish breakouts and clogged pores like the wise Witch you are, harnessing the lunar powers of fruits and herbs to keep skin beautifully clear and bright as stars in the evening sky.

### Ingredients

1 cup blueberries, or 2 teaspoons blueberry powder

6 drops lavender essential oil

3 drops sage essential oil

3 drops lemon essential oil

*Note: If using blueberry powder, add spring water to desired consistency*

**Intention** Acne-fighting, purifying, anti-wrinkle, calming

**Lunar Phase** Waning

**Conjures** 2 treatments

## ᕙ Drench Me, Facial Masque ᕗ

When your face craves major moisture, conjure this: instantly healing, softening, and beautifying, a voluptuous masque that is a delight to use whenever dewy skin has escaped you.

### Ingredients

¼ avocado, very ripe and mashed

1 tablespoon banana, very ripe and mashed, or 1 teaspoon banana powder

1 teaspoon coconut powder

1 teaspoon chia seed oil

3 drops frankincense essential oil

**Intention** Intense moisture, hydration, softens lines, age-defying

**Lunar Phase** Full

**Conjures** 1–2 treatments

# Mystic Chocolat, Facial Masque & Exfoliant

For when only a lusty indulgence will do—a rich, nutritious, reviving facial that lifts away impurities as it infuses skin with bewitching gorgeousness and a scent you will want to devour. Accept this as an offering by the cacao god to the glamour goddess, and revel in its dazzling effects on both your mood and your complexion.

### Ingredients

1 teaspoon raw, unsweetened cacao powder

1 teaspoon almond flour

¼ teaspoon ground cardamom

1 teaspoon almond oil

pinch of cinnamon

**Intention** Polish, firm, nourish, boost circulation

**Lunar Phase** New to full

**Conjures** 1–2 treatments

# Crystal Visions

————•◦▷◆◁◦•————

The beauty of crystals, gems, and sacred stones are amongst the most vivid and intriguing of the magickal realm. Born of the deepest earth, they carry the energies of the land in which they hold court. Like plants, they are varied throughout the world, the carriers of magick specific to their individual climates, planetary rulers, and the richness of minerals present, all woven expertly within ancient tales of mystic ritual.

And they are *gorgeous.* The range of colors and patterns are breathtakingly glamorous—whether atop your altar, carried with you, or resting against your skin—they are aesthetic amazons that dare you to rise to their vibrational caliber.

How about elevating your beauty ritual even higher? Cleansed, charged, and carefully placed, crystals will do sublime things for your skin: lessen fine lines, boost circulation, hydrate, increase elasticity, and so much more. The best part? You get to lie back, adorn your face with stunningly beautiful stones, and *relax.* When you rise, it is with regal grace; rested and refreshed, glowing like one million stars.

Though I would always choose unpolished, raw crystals for altar rituals, those that lie upon your skin should be as smooth and as flat as possible. This allows them to penetrate well by staying put along the contours of your face, without any concern for jagged edges. Try these lunar-aligned combinations, but do create some of your own. Half the fun is in the *play.* And isn't it exuberant to be a kitten sometimes?

## New Moon

*To restore the glow of youth with fresh, energized radiance.*

2 pieces of amber

2 rubies

1 aquamarine

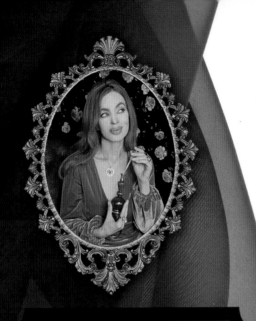

Place one piece of amber on your forehead and chin, one ruby on each cheek, and the aquamarine on your third eye.

## Full Moon

*Age-defying power fit for a Queen.*

2 sapphires

3 emeralds

1 lepidolite

Place the lepidolite on your forehead, one emerald at your third eye and at each corner of the mouth, and one sapphire on each cheek.

## Waning Moon

*To detoxify and heal.*

2 onyx

2 bloodstones

1 shungite

Place one bloodstone each on your forehead and chin, one piece of onyx on each cheek, and the shungite on your third eye.

## ƁEAUTY WITCH SECRET

*How about a quick version that you can do every day? If you have never used a crystal facial roller, you are in for a treat! Though commonly found in jade (which, of course, holds its own unique powers,) I like to seek out ones made of rose quartz, which brings not only a vital beauty energy, but also a certain lightness that's just lovely on your face. Apply a beauty oil to clean skin, then roll in upward strokes beginning from the neck, and continuing all the way to the top of the forehead. For extra de-puffing prowess, store in the freezer and use ice cold.*

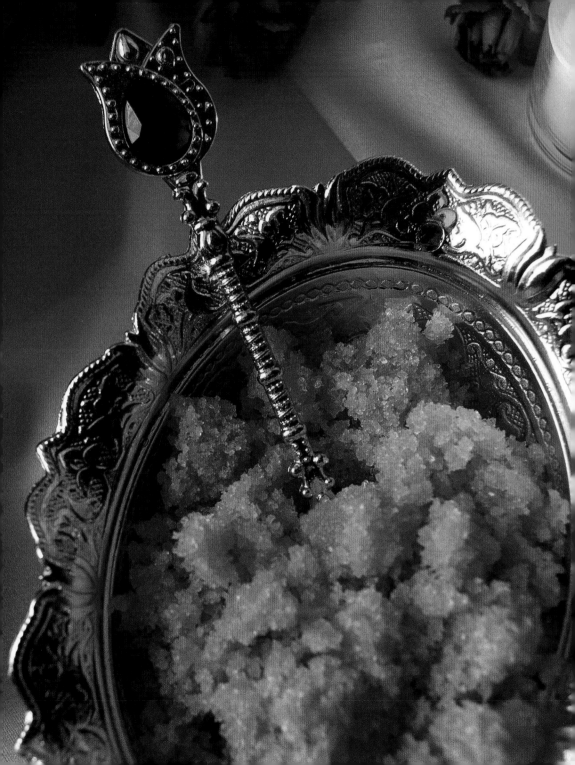

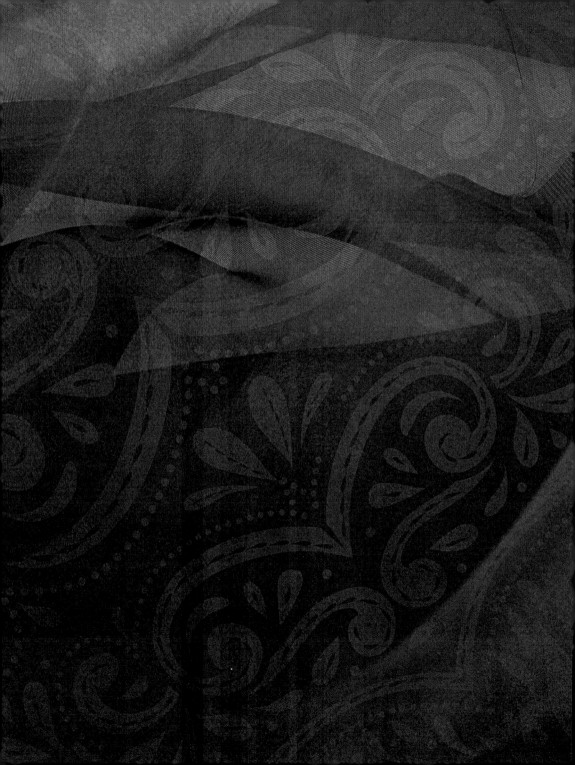

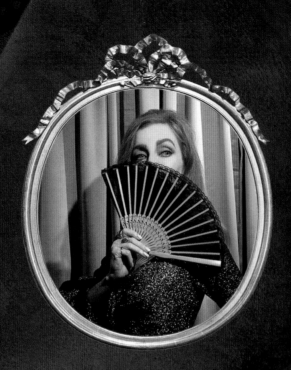

## Chapter Seven
# The Female Gaze

The windows of the soul offer not only a peek behind the curtain of the possessor, should she deign to allow it, but also hold a unique power to bewitch. At once expressive and entirely seductive, they glimmer with delight, flare with passion, and dance with joy. Then on a dime they turn cool and distant, in a fixed, unwavering veneer that dares the beholder to guess their secrets.

The female gaze, when she is in in her full power, is akin to the unblinking stare of a cat: a silent channeling of affection, granted only when this mysterious creature feels safe and secure. The otherworldly glance, the hypnotic beauty of the eyes fixating on its subject, or perhaps seeing right through it, never ceases to beguile.

Handle with extra care these gorgeous transmitters of emotion, whether sharing an intimate moment with a lover, a wink with a co-worker, or a giggle with a friend, remember: the eyes of a wise Witch always enchant.

# The Ritual of the Eyes

When stirred from slumber each morning, the eyes require a moment to flutter awake. Potions are summoned to soothe, tighten, and brighten to greet the new day with the gaze of youth, bright and ready for action! In the evening, as we prepare for beauty sleep, richer concoctions are summoned to work their magick in the resting hours, undisturbed, as the body regenerates itself.

### Cleanse

A light, gentle tap of makeup remover (Strip Tease, p. 83–84) delicately massaged into the lashes effectively cleanses all traces of cosmetics, and will even remove evidence of the sandman's visit when you wake. Beauty Witch bonus: regular use will build long, silky lashes, and help to fill in sparse brows.

### Anoint

Dab 1–2 drops of potion onto your ring finger, then share it with the other hand by tapping it onto the opposite ring finger. Begin to tap lightly into the bone just *below* the eye, known as the orbital bone. Do not rub or massage into the skin, and avoid the very delicate area just beneath your eye. This is important—you can easily create wrinkles and sagging skin by rubbing or tugging too hard. When you tap gently along the orbital bone, the oils will absorb *up* into the fine skin. You can also tap it along the bone under your brow (supraorbital) to de-puff and firm that area also. Finish by fluttering all your fingertips around the eye bones, just as you did on your face, like stardust being sprinkled!

Adorn

As with all beauty potions, only use clean makeup worthy of your fabulous gaze. Cruelty-free, nourishing, eco-friendly makeup has come such a long way in recent years, so finding that fantastic shade or texture is completely within reach. See the Resources section (p. 235) for companies that have high standards and knockout products.

## The Maiden's Gaze, Beauty Oil

Use daily during your morning ritual, inhaling the heady scents and exotic atmosphere of sipping a Turkish coffee in the Grand Bazaar. Magickal bonus: frankincense lifts vibrations as well as sagging skin, to begin your day with bright optimism and unfaltering confidence.

### Ingredients

1 oz. rosehip oil

1 oz. almond oil

1 tablespoon finely ground organic coffee (espresso grind)

13 drops frankincense oil

3 drops sandalwood oil

## BEAUTY WITCH SECRET

*Sleepy eyes? Douse a facial pad with a bit of rosewater, close your eyes, and apply. Let it sit for a minute to absorb into the skin. When you open your eyes, they will feel awake and moisturized. This is wonderful first thing in the morning after cleansing to clear any traces of sleep and open your vision to the possibilities of the day.*

1 tablespoon pure coffee extract

½ teaspoon amber resin, crushed to powder

1 small piece of amber

**Intention** Brighten, tighten, hydrate, soothe

**Lunar Phase** New

**Conjures** 1–2 month supply

## The Feline Stare, Eye Gel

Dab this sparingly as part of your evening ritual before retiring. Its richness will have time to absorb into your skin as you sleep, while its lusciousness lulls you to the sweetest dreamtime.

This also makes a gorgeous spa treatment, when you have time to allow it to really drink into your skin—it has the delightful scent and texture of lemon chiffon—before an event or a glittering evening out, ensuring the tiger's eyes are at their most enchanting.

### Ingredients

½ teaspoon sweet almond oil

½ teaspoon vitamin E oil

1 teaspoon cucumber extract

1 teaspoon green tea extract

2 tablespoons pure aloe vera gel

½ teaspoon ginseng extract

8 drops lemon essential oil

**Intention** Firm, tighten, revitalize, hydrate, soothe, brighten

**Lunar Phase** New

**Conjures** 2–3 month supply

# Bisous des Yeux, Eye Mist

When those bedroom eyes become unbearably heavy, this delightful potion will brighten them right up! Be it a light mid-day mist atop your makeup, or spritzed on cotton pads while reclining *sans maquillage*, this blend soothes and cools irritated peepers, restoring that mesmerizing Bast gaze to its full power.

### Ingredients

2 oz. spring water

1 tablespoon chamomile flowers

1 teaspoon green tea extract

1 teaspoon cucumber extract

1 piece lapis lazuli

**Intention** Refresh, revive, soothe

**Lunar Phase** New

**Conjures** 2 month supply

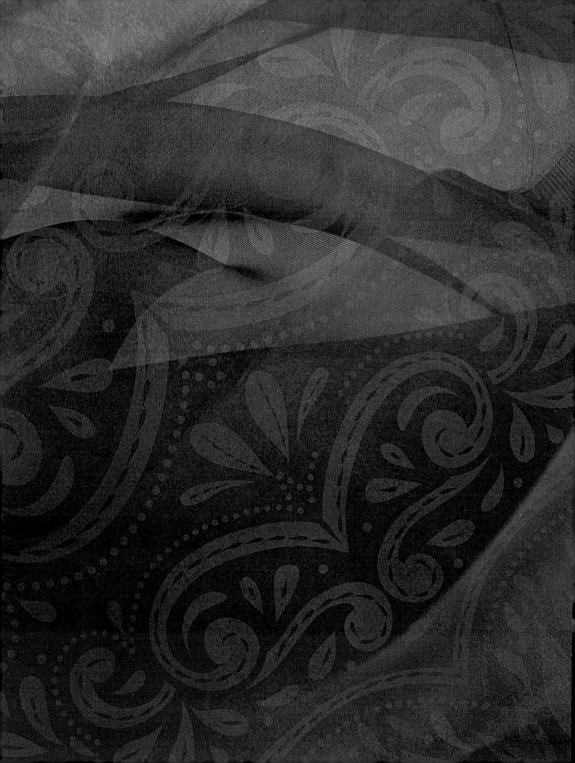

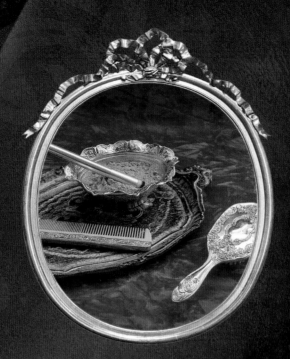

Chapter Eight

# Crowning Glory

A Witch's mane is indeed her Crown of Stars, with cosmic threads woven through each strand by the element of air. Flirtatious and coy, hair conveys sexuality and sensuality perhaps even more than any other part of us when left in a touchable state. Think of classic Bardot, with her soft curls, obviously done, but then left to be free and charmingly tousled, as if she has always just emerged from a secret, delightful tryst. Loose or adorned, a good hair day bestows confidence like no other, so the aim here is to conjure salon-sexy magnificence every day. No matter what your personal style, be it long or short, straight or curly, conservative or wild, this lightness of being is beyond alluring, and best achieved by taking exquisite care of your fine feathers.

A tumble of tresses that frames your exquisite face is not only coveted, but holds energy—*your* energy, be it positive or negative—and that energy accumulates. As such, regular brushing, massaging, and even a ritual smoke cleanse is as much a necessity as feeding and conditioning. This keeps the crown chakra open, allowing access to higher states of consciousness. And don't neglect those essential visits to your stylist during a waning moon; a good chop will keep the old energy from hanging on, as well as ensuring healthy hair that always holds its shape. Trying a new shade? Do it when the moon is waxing—but be sure to come prepared with visuals and a realistic sense of your texture, coloring, and facial structure. And now, behold the tried and true secrets of maintaining your mane, and unleash that which has beguiled for centuries: the witchcraft that lies within your tendrils.

# The Ritual of the Hair

## Cleanse

The simple act of shampooing can be either mundane of magickal, the latter of which is attained by elevating the act to that of ritual. You are not simply *washing your hair*, my felines, you are banishing old energy, energy that is currently weighing down your entire being without you even knowing it. It is also weighing down your mane, so let us be done with it! How often you shampoo is up to your hair, really, but ideally not something you do every single day. Why? Because hair's natural oils protect it. You don't want to strip that away, but nor do you want a buildup of dirt, oil, and product to sit on your scalp forever—this can cause hair growth to slow, even to a grinding halt. Enjoying a fresh mane then giving it a rest for a day (or more, if you can) is a favorable cycle, gently brushing through to bring those oils from the scalp to the ends, and giving it all a delicious little massage in the process, letting go of the old and preparing for the new. And for really doing a little energetic exorcism, try this: during a waning-to-dark moon, light a sage or mugwort bundle, bend down and flip your hair over, then *carefully* allow the smoke to waft up into your strands, using your fingers to help it penetrate throughout. It's also a lovely thing to do for someone else, and have done to you by a trusted confidante.

## Feed

Your hair and scalp are two different creatures, one essentially feeding the other. When healthy, your scalp acts as a mama cat nourishing all her little tendril kittens, giving them everything they need to grow strong and resilient. In order to do this, the scalp needs excellent circulation and a steady absorption of vitamins, minerals, and fortifying herbs. Treat her to not only regular conditioning, but also specialized masques to vitalize and deeply condition, particularly during a growing moon.

## Arrange

Styling can be such a fickle thing. Ideally, a great cut precludes having to do anything, but how often is this actually the case? The days are few and far between where we can simply shake our mane and go, so some degree of styling magick is usually in order. Try to keep heat appliances and back combing to a minimum (but if you insist, there's a potion waiting for you on p. 108.) I'm a firm believer in having a few "be kind to your hair" days per week where you let your tresses have a rest by coating your ends with a little conditioning oil or crème, then curling it all up into a simple updo. Hats and scarves are employed in a similar fashion, minus the oil (usually.) For heat-free bombshell waves, mist sections with floral water (lavender is excellent,) curl around two or three fingers, and secure with a clip. Let it set for at least 30 minutes—the longer the better—then unclip and let the waves tumble down. Comb through with fingers or gently with a brush, and prepare to bewitch.

## Protect

A crowning coat of armor is vital to hair's resilience. Environmental stress, heat appliances, weather, indoor air, and even precious sunlight can wreak havoc on our manes. A protective force field against anything that dares damage your strands is essential. In cold months, always keep a scarf handy to wrap around your head, movie-star style. Besides being mysterious, it will protect your hair from the ravages of weaving in and out of dry indoor air and the frigid outdoors when the hair strands expand and contract constantly, making them highly susceptible to breakage. As you prepare for beauty sleep, mist ends lightly, perhaps dabbing the ends just a bit with conditioning oil or crème, then securing a chignon high atop your head with rubber-tipped hair pins or a stretchy band (no elastic!)

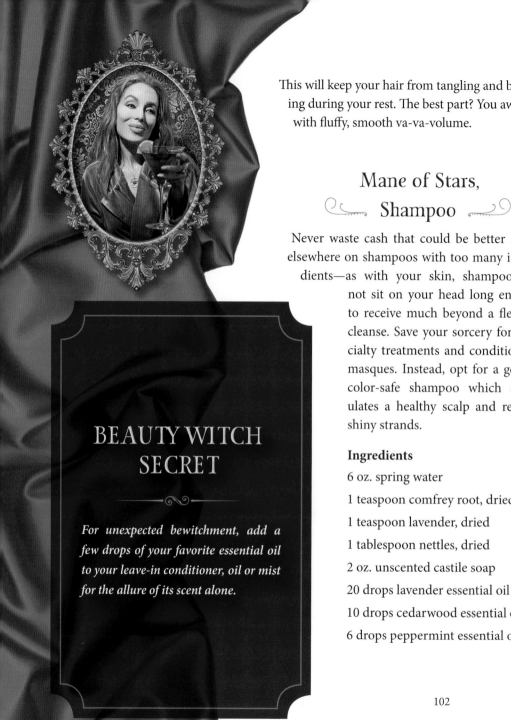

This will keep your hair from tangling and breaking during your rest. The best part? You awaken with fluffy, smooth va-va-volume.

## Mane of Stars, Shampoo

Never waste cash that could be better spent elsewhere on shampoos with too many ingredients—as with your skin, shampoos do not sit on your head long enough to receive much beyond a fleeting cleanse. Save your sorcery for specialty treatments and conditioning masques. Instead, opt for a gentle, color-safe shampoo which stimulates a healthy scalp and reveals shiny strands.

### Ingredients

6 oz. spring water

1 teaspoon comfrey root, dried

1 teaspoon lavender, dried

1 tablespoon nettles, dried

2 oz. unscented castile soap

20 drops lavender essential oil

10 drops cedarwood essential oil

6 drops peppermint essential oil

## BEAUTY WITCH SECRET

*For unexpected bewitchment, add a few drops of your favorite essential oil to your leave-in conditioner, oil or mist for the allure of its scent alone.*

**Intention** Cleanse, boost circulation, promote hair growth

**Lunar Phase** New

**Conjures** 1 month supply

## Silken Threads, Conditioner

Treat your tresses to a conditioner that leaves them soft, shiny, and easily managed—but never weighed down. Moisture is locked, your hair is loaded. With magick to conjure growth and thickness, let's just say your hair will adore you. Just follow the instructions for making crèmes (p. 48–50) to concoct your very own Secret Hair Weapon. And when they ask," What conditioner are you using? Your hair is gorgeous!" you flash a Cheshire smile and simply say, "Oh, just a little potion I whipped up."

### Ingredients
**Phase One**

1½ oz. shea butter

½ oz. candelilla wax

3 oz. avocado oil

**Phase Two**

4 oz. spring water

**Phase Three**

20 drops lavender essential oil

10 drops jasmine essential oil

**Intention** Moisture, shine, softness

**Lunar Phase** Waxing

**Conjures** 1–2 month supply

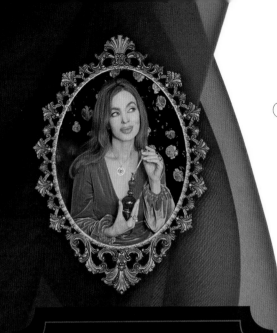

# Luscious Locks, Hair Masque

If, despite your best efforts, you should find your mane parched and unhappy, rescue it immediately with this intensive repair potion. Deep conditioning and glorious shine are restored, hair is protected from the evils of breakage, and you are once again ready to bewitch with a toss of your head.

**Ingredients**

½ very ripe avocado

2 tablespoon Abyssinian oil

1 teaspoon licorice root

1 teaspoon comfrey, dried

1 teaspoon elder flowers, dried and crushed

**Intention** Restore, protect, deep condition

**Lunar Phase** New to full

**Conjures** One treatment

## BEAUTY WITCH SECRET

*Use a drop of Silken Threads as a leave-in conditioner, and leave a breath of intoxicating scent wherever you go.*

## ⟿ Lady of the Golden Wood, Hair Masque ⟿

Named for the Lady Galadriel's glorious, glimmering tresses, this potion calls in immortal Elven beauty. It lavishes your hair with nutritive oils that deeply moisturize, strengthen, and promote new growth to your mane, while keeping it light and full of life. Use this to restore hair any time you like. It is particularly effective during the new-to-full moon cycle.

### Ingredients

½ banana, very ripe and mashed

1 tablespoon grapeseed oil

6 drops lavender essential oil

3 drops rosemary essential oil

4 drops ylang ylang essential oil

**Intention** Restore, strengthen, impart shine, new growth

**Lunar Phase** New to full

**Conjures** 1–2 treatments

## ⟿ The Polished Crown, Hair Masque ⟿

When your highly important scalp gets cranky and irritable, give it some love with this healing potion concocted to banish itch, dandruff, and inflammation. A slow, sensual massage will lift away what ails you as it infuses herbal charms to restore regal grace and tranquility.

**Ingredients**

2 tablespoons coconut oil

1 teaspoon vitamin E oil

9 drops lavender essential oil

6 drops thyme essential oil

6 drops cypress essential oil

**Intention** Relieve irritated & flaky scalp, soothe, heal

**Lunar Phase** Waning

**Conjures** One treatment

# Follicle Frolic, Hair Rinse

Give your crowning glory a joyous refresher with a rinse that vanquishes product buildup and lingering energy as it feeds the scalp with stimulating, nutritive treasures. Après shampoo, pour this potion slowly onto your head and onto hair, massaging in sensually, and allowing it to sit a moment, breathing in its sexy scent. Rinse with cool water, and seal it with a bit of conditioner for bouncy, shiny, well-fed locks. I like to perform this ritual once during the waning cycle, and again on the new moon.

**Ingredients**

¼ cup apple cider vinegar, unfiltered

¼ cup spring water

13 drops cedarwood essential oil

6 drops nutmeg essential oil

6 drops ylang ylang essential oil

**Intention** Clarify, balance pH, shine

**Lunar Phase** New

**Conjures** One treatment

## The Lion's Roar, Hair Volumizer

This blend gives an amazing lift to your mane, and can also be used as a fantastic dry shampoo. Simply blend together and apply to root area in sections using a cosmetic brush, then massage in with your fingers. The powdered texture absorbs excess oil, while the nutmeg actually infuses the scalp and hair with its own nutritive oil, a timeless secret to actually growing hair! Have fun with this anytime you need your hair to be its most buxom, and especially leading up to, and during, the full moon, when Jupiter-ruled nutmeg can help you tap into your third eye to help you manifest your wishes.

**Ingredients**

¼ cup arrowroot powder

¼ cup ground nutmeg

**Intention** Volume, growth, protection,

**Lunar Phase** New to full

**Conjures** 2–3 month supply

# Tendril Tamer, Hair Mist

This light, lustrous potion is an all-around magickal hair mist: it hydrates and moisturizes without oiliness, detangles, imparts starlight shine, calms frizzies, protects from heat damage and even offers a bit of UV protection. Mist it on whenever your mane needs refreshing—it works well on all textures.

**Ingredients**

1½ oz. rose water

3 drops rosehip oil

1 teaspoon Abyssinian oil

3 drops avocado oil

1 teaspoon vegetable glycerin

**Intention** Shine, detangle, protect

**Lunar Phase** Full

**Conjures** 1–2 month supply

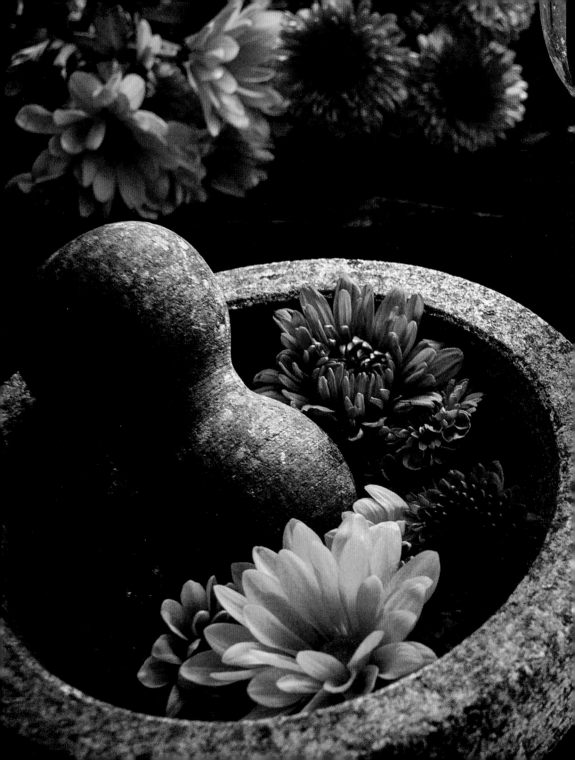

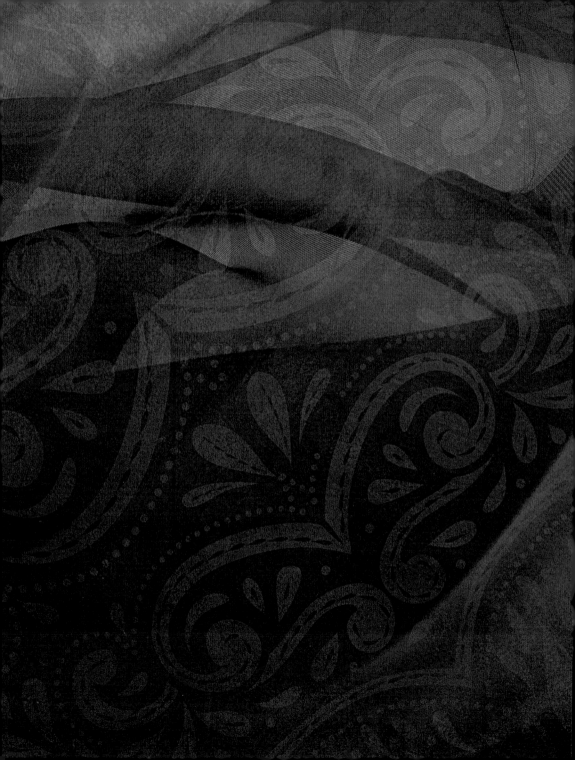

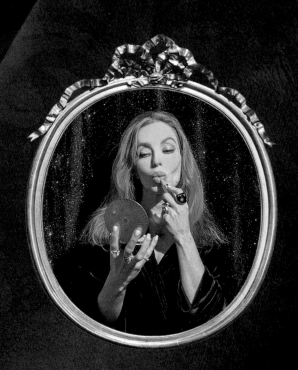

## Chapter Nine

# The Witch's Kiss

The lips, like lusciously ripe fruit, are best enjoyed when bitten at just the right moment. Brushed lightly to arouse, nibbled, then ultimately devoured, the mouth is an exquisite erogenous zone that has many powers beyond the obvious. Through it we enchant with song, whisper sweet nothings, speak our minds, purr with delight, embrace the flesh of lovers, smile radiantly, laugh uproariously, and moan in ecstasy. The mouth, indeed, deserves a very special place of honor upon the altar of beauty.

A flower of many soft petals, drenched in honeyed nectar, and always the exact shade of allure, it opens to reveal glistening pearls. The teeth, gleaming, convey joy and grace as easily as an angry hiss. The tongue savors salty skin as willingly as it does the ambrosia of fresh berries. The voice, always commanding, modulates between a soft coo and an emphatic roar, depending on which Witch you are in that moment. Honor your beautiful *bouche* with tantalizing potions and prized rituals, and prepare to hold all in your sway.

# The Ritual of the Kiss

## Purify

Delectable smooches and fascinating conversations begin with breath that beckons. The root of fresh breath begins with digestion, so pop some papaya enzymes before each meal, and nibble a sprig of mint, or even parsley, whenever possible après feast. Use natural whitening and cleaning potions that support healthy teeth and gums, and always carry a bottle of food-grade peppermint oil in your handbag for a quick breath freshener. You can drop a little right on your tongue, or into your water bottle, and rinse—instant magick mouthwash!

## Polish

A Witch will never tolerate less-than-sumptuous lips, so a good exfoliation needs to happen daily, and even more frequently in dry weather. Sloughing off chapped skin plumps and smooths lines by circulating the blood, revealing a fuller, softer pout. Begin your daily beauty ritual with an exfoliating potion (See Purrfect Pout, p. 115) and use this trick for lush lips on the go: slick on a bit of balm or beauty oil, then massage vigorously with a travel toothbrush, kept on hand exclusively for pout perfection. Wipe clean, then apply your favorite lipstick for newly revived, entirely come-hither lips that invite endless *bisous*.

## Infuse

Just as chapped skin can rob your lips of their inherent charms, so can the underlying dryness. Dehydrated mouths look unwell, and feel awful. Drench your lips in rich, hydrating moisture as often as they need it with potions specifically crafted with your mouth in mind. Left your lip balm at home? Lightly apply facial moisturizers, oils, or even hand crème—they'll do in a pinch. The important thing is to lock in hydration, which begins with the most basic tenet of bewitching beauty: drink water. Oh, you do? That's wonderful. *Now drink more.*

## Anoint

And at last, the cherry on top: lipstick. The name alone conjures images of succulent fruits, and with it the instant confidence boost that a simple swathe of sublime color can give. It is the quickest possible mood lifter and look-polisher there is. Oh, and the shades! One for every mood, every season, every outfit! The smart witch avoids those of the nasty, chemical laden variety though (yes, it can be a challenge) and opts instead for clean, natural lipsticks that nourish and protect lips instead of robbing them, ultimately, of their much-needed moisture. Oh that, and the fact that we choose not to ingest said chemicals into our bodies.

# Baume Bisou, Lip Balm

The finishing touch to your sorceress' smooch—a beautifying balm to anoint your lips with plush moisture that absorbs easily as it assists in collagen production. Excellent as a sensual base for your favorite lipstick, or flaunt au naturel. If you're feeling especially romantic, add a teaspoon of rose-colored mica powder for a just-bitten tint.

**Ingredients**

**Phase One**

1 oz. avocado oil

1 oz. rosehip oil

1 oz. candelilla wax

**Phase Three**

1 teaspoon hyaluronic acid

1 vanilla bean, seeded

16 drops rose absolute

**Intention** Softening, collagen building, hydrating, protective

**Lunar Phase** Waxing to full

**Conjures** 3–6 month supply

## Kiss Me, Tooth Polish

Seductive smiles can lead to so much more … heighten the electricity with a two-step ritual for star-powered pearly whites: Use the coconut oil blend on your toothbrush as you would commercial toothpaste for everyday dazzle, then follow by brushing with the baking soda twice weekly for megawatt allure. Your dentist and your lover will be impressed.

**Ingredients**

2 tablespoons coconut oil

1 teaspoon turmeric

20 drops peppermint essential oil

20 drops clove essential oil

8 drops tea tree essential oil

2 tablespoons baking soda

*Note: Store oil blend and baking soda in two separate containers*

**Intention** Cleanse, strengthen gums, whiten, freshen

**Lunar Phase** Waning

**Conjures** 1 month supply

## Purrfect Pout, Exfoliant

Pucker up, baby. No dry, dehydrated, chapped kisses will be tolerated. Keep your pout plumped and ready for anything with this potion that casts a kaleidoscopic spell: it lifts away dead skin cells while it repairs lips, stimulates circulation for fullness, adds nourishment and seals in rich moisture. *Bisous* à *vous!*

**Ingredients**

1 tablespoon coconut oil

1 teaspoon avocado oil

½ teaspoon hyaluronic acid

¼ teaspoon vitamin E oil

1 tablespoon raw coconut sugar

1 teaspoon ground ginger

1 teaspoon ground cayenne

**Intention** Exfoliate, soften, plump

**Lunar Phase** New

**Conjures** 30 treatments

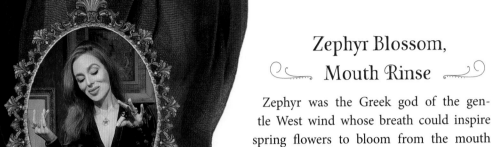

# Zephyr Blossom,
## Mouth Rinse

Zephyr was the Greek god of the gentle West wind whose breath could inspire spring flowers to bloom from the mouth of a nymph. Inspired by his tale, this potion bestows beautiful breath that might just open the door to a budding new adventure. Concoct an extra batch in a spray bottle, and toss it in your handbag—you never know when you might cross paths with sultry stranger.

**Ingredients**

3 oz. spring water

40 drops peppermint essential oil

20 drops clove essential oil

10 drops nutmeg essential oil

**Intention** Freshen, banish germs, soothe

**Lunar phase** New

**Conjures** 15 treatments

## BEAUTY WITCH SECRET

*A dab of hydrating facial masque around the mouth in between treatments provides instant plumping for those pesky kissy lines, as does a regular wave of the magick (high-frequency) wand.*

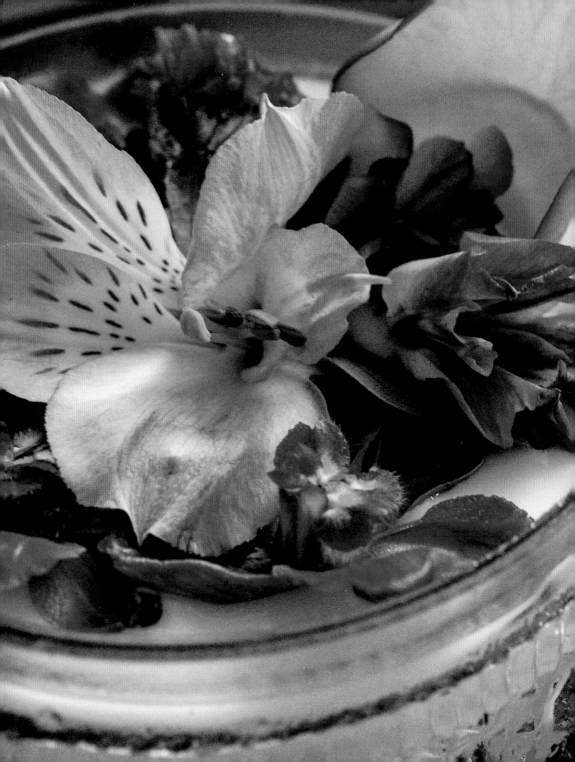

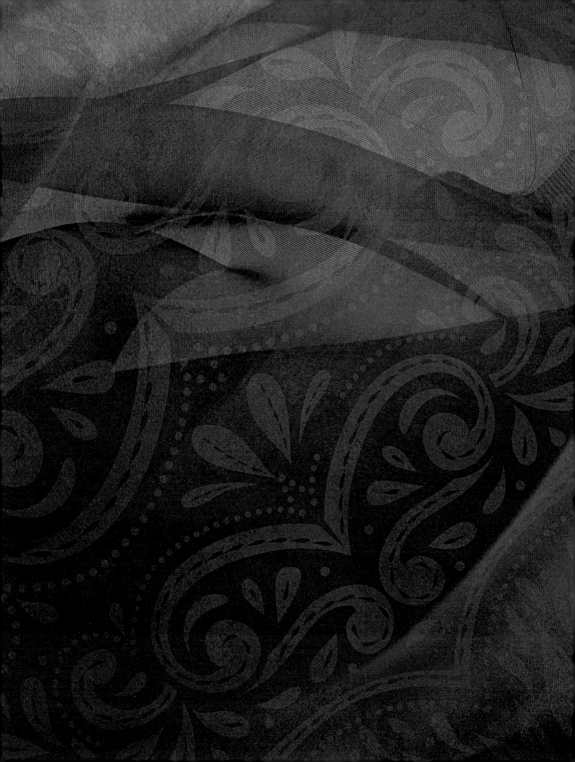

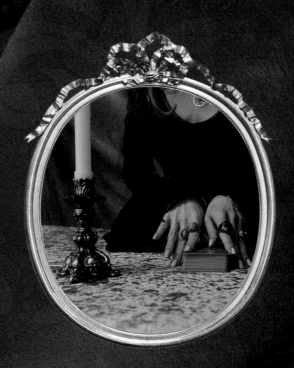

Chapter Ten

# Hands of Fate

The delicate fingers that draw sense though touch are the very same wands that cast spells, weaving magick throughout everything you choose to create. They are the conductors of both giving and receiving sensual caresses, and those with which you touch your own flesh in beauty ritual, every single day. They are the hands of the artist that bring into existence what was before only a thought, and then, through the enchantment of touch, becomes a work of substance. Resourceful and multitalented, they know just how to expertly stroke a lover, bring much-needed comfort to a child, and calmly reassure an animal of your kindness. Whether tending a garden that comes alive with the magick of plant power or penning a sweet note to a loved one, our precious paws are forever communicating.

Similar to the feet, the hands are often fetishized, though not to the same extent. Rings are symbolic of love, prosperity, and the passions of the individual. Gloves, though now worn mostly for warmth, are still in certain circles added as a finishing touch to an ensemble, on steamy occasions becoming an accessory of bewitching eroticism. Nails are obsessively groomed, often with more attention paid to them than to the rest of the body, by way of the Stateside national pastime—the manicure.

I'm going to let you in on a little secret: tending your hands at home is incredibly sexy. As I've said, there is nothing quite like casting a spell upon yourself with beauty rituals at home, and this is no exception. Think about it—you are infusing with sorcery the very tools of *your* trade. In the sanctity of your own space, filled with all your uniquely spell-binding mojo, you are preparing, raising energy, and sending them out into the world as ambassadors of your magick.

# The Ritual of the Hands

## Cleanse

It's only really necessary to cleanse what actually touches things, sparing the rest from being stripped of precious oils, especially because hands require more frequent washing to protect the entire body from germs. The oft-forgotten hands have the unfortunate distinction of showing age more quickly than the face, so focus cleansing on fingertips, palms, and under nails, sparing the back of hands from over-drying. A good nail brush does wonders for removing bacteria, especially with longer claws, and it feels fabulous.

## Exfoliate

Oh yes. Hands need constant care, and the best way to prepare them for moisture is by sloughing. Every time you use gentle exfoliant on your face and neck, include your hands—I promise you will begin to see a difference. When you use a body scrub, don't forget paws! The rich oils will penetrate after the old cells are removed, making them look better than they have in a while. The same goes for peels. Keep up the ritual, and the results will be cumulative.

## Cloak

Hands crave a protective veil just as the rest of the body. Beauty Witch Rule: *Never go near dishes or a powder room tidying without wearing gloves. Never.* Housework gloves save your hands and nails from a disastrous fate, make no mistake, and you can actually find some fetching ones out there. In fact, wear gloves for everything! Soft, warm ones to protect from the harsh winds, lacy little ones out on the town, and opera length bomb-shells to really make a statement. When left to frolic uncovered, do your hands the favor of wearing sunscreen, and I do mean always. Age spots will never be confused with those of a leopard, so we have no use for them.

## Drench

Your hands can never have enough hydration, so moisturize like mad. Extend your daily beauty oil and crème anointing to include the hands, and keep a little jar of potion everywhere—your handbag, at work, in the car, sink side in the kitchen, and atop the bedside table. Use your softening and anti-aging facial masques as spa treatments when-ever you indulge your face and neck, liberally coating the back of hands and fingers. It may require a little extra attention to get into the habit, but it's beyond worth it. Try cot-ton gloves, too, for deep overnight moisturizing. (When you are sleeping alone, that is.)

## Adorn

At last we arrive at the fun part! Decorating the talons is so pleasurable, especially when we take it upon ourselves as part of a beauty ritual. There is an innate sensuality in lacquering our nails—perhaps it's the sweeping strokes, the color that comes alive, the glossy finishing touches, who knows? Maybe it's all of them, and the moments we take to admire them languidly as they dry, ideally with a glass of bubbly in hand. Opt for only clean polish—often called "5-free" or even up to "12-free," mean-ing free of the most common toxins—to steer clear of drying (not to mention potentially dangerous) chemicals, and take a day off at least once weekly to allow the nails to breathe. A good file is essential—have you tried the frosted glass ones yet? They're fantastic. File in one direction to keep nails strong, and keep one in your handbag for unexpected snags. Massaging oils into the cuticle and nail regularly helps immensely too.

## Magick Touch, Hand Mist

Oh, those little dirt goblins that seem to be everywhere! Pesky creatures, prepare to be banished by the magick of plants that mingle within this sexy Witches version of the unappealingly named "hand sanitizer." This potion smells gorgeous and powerful, because it is. Spray on hands whenever the situation is less than savory, and give germs the pointy boot.

**Ingredients**

2½ oz. spring water

13 drops clove essential oil

9 drops cinnamon essential oil

6 drops thyme essential oil

6 drops wild orange essential oil

6 drops grapefruit essential oil

*Note: 120-proof vodka can be used in place of spring water if needed.*

**Intention** Disinfect, cleanse, protect

**Lunar Phase** Waning

**Conjures** 1–2 month supply

## ⌒ Polished Paws, Exfoliant ⌒

Velvety soft kitten's paws may seem agonizingly out of reach, but actually, they can be captured quite easily with a bit of mindful maintenance. A good sloughing every other day, followed by additional moisture and protection, will begin to transform them from ancient artifacts to the elegant beasts they truly are.

### Ingredients

1 cup brown rice flour

¾ cup grapeseed oil

1 tablespoon vitamin E oil

6 drops sandalwood essential oil

1 small rough-cut emerald

**Intention** Exfoliate, renew, protect, heal

**Lunar Phase** New

**Conjures** 8 treatments

## ⌒ Velvet Glove, Hand & Nail Oil ⌒

For comely claws and tantalizing talons, anoint your hands, cuticles and nail bed with this potion every chance you get—even if you are sporting lacquer, the nourishing oil will massage in, ensuring healthy new growth and hands that beckon fine jewels be placed upon each finger.

### Ingredients

2 oz. sweet almond oil

1 teaspoon vitamin E oil

6 drops lavender

6 drops lemon

10 drops myrrh

1 small piece of lapis lazuli

**Intention** Repair, protect, prevent peeling and breakage, strengthen

**Lunar Phase** New to full

**Conjures** 2–3 month supply

## Let Me Read Your Palm, Hand Crème

"Ah, yes … I see you have a very deep love line." The finishing touch for your pretty paws involves high-powered plant magick for richly hydrated skin and wrinkles kept firmly at bay, giving you the softest touch in town. You'll have them eating right out of your hand.

### Ingredients
### Phase One

⅓ cup cacao butter

¼ cup meadowfoam seed oil

¼ cup borage oil

¼ cup avocado oil

1 tablespoon candelilla wax

### Phase Two

⅔ cup rosewater

⅓ cup aloe vera gel

**Phase Three**

1 teaspoon hyaluronic acid

20 drops frankincense essential oil

10 drops lemon essential oil

**Intention** Deep moisture, hydration, protection, lightens hyperpigmentation, anti-aging

**Lunar Phase** Full

**Conjures** 13 oz.

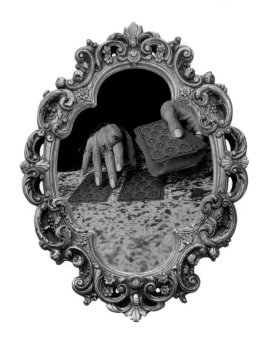

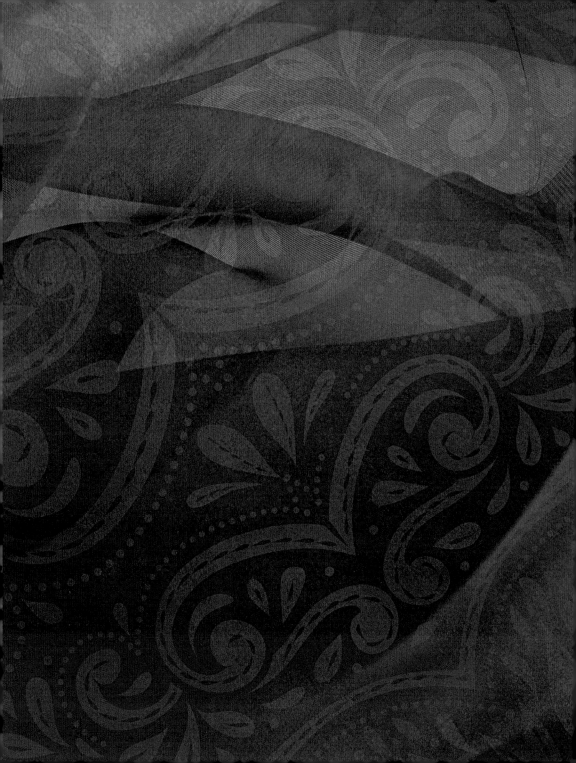

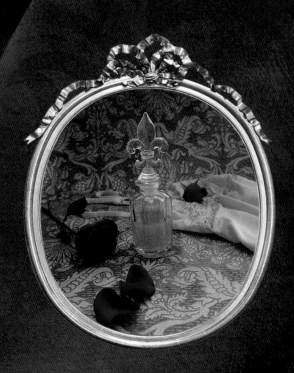

## Chapter Eleven

# Your Heavenly Body

**Y**our body is the blessed temple which shelters your divine essence of spirit, housing your ever-burning internal fire. But is it a fire, really, that you are continually stoking, allowing the flame to glow brightly, or in the clutches of daily life has this magnificent blaze been reduced to ash? Beauties, that fire can build again. And it can smolder continually with bombshell vibrancy. The ritual of reclaiming begins with a commitment to *loving* your body.

It is the literal expression of sensuality we are gifted with, and yet, too often, we leave this sacred space unattended. Perhaps we do not see its true beauty, but rather as a vehicle for dragging from place to place—a notion which brings tears to the eyes of the sensual Witch. After all, what is a temple, but a house of worship? That which you direct your focus upon blossoms, while that which we ignore withers. This is the doctrine of the earthy goddess in her garden, but also the basics of how energy works, and thus, Magick 101.

It is not a luxury to stimulate your skin with crystalline pearls that uncover, nor to caress it with precious dew, releasing intoxicating scents and draping your entire being in moonglow. *It is sacrosanct.* It is the act of worshipping at the altar of your own well-being. And though our faces are the calling cards of our physicality, our bodies do us the favor of transporting us wherever we wish to be, unleashing our carnal desires, and undulating with the rhythm of the oceans. How can we ever thank such a magnificent machine? By honoring her as the divine creature she is.

# The Five-Fold Kiss

Traditional Witchcraft bestows the ritual of The Five-Fold Kiss upon the High Priestess by the High Priest (or vice-versa) by kneeling before her naked body to bless and worship her from her feet all the way up to her brow or crown chakra, depending on the observances of each individual coven. A line of prayer is said as her body is kissed each at the feet, the knees, the womb, the breasts and the lips—often omitting the knees in favor of the 3rd eye or the top of the head. Some older traditions even observed the Six- or Seven-Fold Kiss, so as to get the entire body in!

Why not incorporate this into your daily ritual? Giving thanks to the body is something we tend to tragically overlook. Holding the body in high esteem *just as it is right now* is as powerful a tool as visualizing what you would like it to become. And you know where it works especially well? On those bits and bobs we aren't so crazy about. It's easy, really, to give your body some appreciation during an *après*-bath application of a favorite oil or crème on, say, something as inoffensive as your feet. But what happens when you get to your not-so-beloved thighs or belly? Off we go, right into self-loathing. But we are Witches, and we are here not only to affect change, but to empower ourselves—that means *every* inch. Now, understand that is not an act of delusion, blindly accepting that which we are unhappy with or may be affecting our good health, but rather a way of giving those less-than-fabulous areas a warm embrace, thanking them for the service they perform every single day for us. You may not love your legs, but they get you where you need to go. Obsessing about jiggly arms? Remember that they carry and cradle your babies (fur or otherwise) in safety. Wish your breasts were different somehow, be it larger, smaller, or firmer? They represent your heart and feed your young, and *especially* need your appreciation for their continued good health. You catch my drift here. Every part of your blessed temple is to be valued.

Try this: when you are done bathing or showering, choose the most appropriate moisturizing potion from this chapter to suit your need, and massage it in, beginning at your feet. As you softly knead, thank them for faithfully, *constantly* taking you places, supporting your entire body, and for putting up with your penchant for heels. (You may even wish to sweet-talk them a bit here, something along the lines of how gorgeous they look in said heels, especially those vintage ankle straps you just snagged for a song.) Now continue on up, all the way to your head. When you hit a spot you aren't crazy about, just find the positive aspect, such as the actual function of that body part, and gently give it some much-needed love. Here's where you can whisper your plans for how to make that area even better, sending that energy out into the cosmos simply by acknowledging it in a sweet way.

Sound complicated? It's not. It needn't take more than a few minutes, and trust me, *mes amours,* you will feel amazing afterward. You have made a sacred pact with your body to love and honor it, and it will in turn do the same.

## The Ritual of the Body

If you are a stranger to body worship, there is no time like the present to begin a daily ritual. If you are seasoned, now is the moment to begin to sprinkle some weekly and monthly stardust on top for extra wattage.

## Cleanse

It all begins with purifying your pores and clearing your energetic space. Whether you favor a sudsy soap or a creamy cleanser, only gentle will do, regardless of skin type. Ingredients high in nutrients, and often high in price, are wasted here, as cleanser does not stay on the skin long enough to be absorbed to any real efficacy. Keep it simple, and only use on those areas which actually get dirty to avoid over-drying. And always rinse thoroughly to remove residue, which can clog pores.

## Exfoliate

Though best done during the waning-to-dark moon phase, gently sloughing away old skin cells can be done as part of your weekly beauty ceremonies. This will help to keep circulation moving, by increasing blood flow and aiding in release of toxins. Besides, it feels *incredible*. As with the face, though, the new skin on your body after shedding the old layer becomes vulnerable, so feed it with nutritive oils and crèmes, and be sure to wear sunscreen outside. A very pleasurable plan would be to use a dry brush weekly, then upgrade to a scrub a few times during the Waning cycle. Remember that shaving is also a form of exfoliation, so be sure to heed the needs of your gorgeous gams and give them a little extra hydration.

## Moisturize

Now, be honest, how often do you scrimp on body moisture? While we obsessively tend to our faces, everything below the chin is nearly forgotten in a hasty attempt to get dressed and out the door. But a quick slather of lotion simply will not do. The body needs rich, nutritive plant foods just as our faces do, and need not succumb to aging poorly. Trust me when I tell you, sexy Witches, that your skin *can* stay incredibly soft, smooth, firm and supple well into your years as you frolic unabashedly, bare limbs to the sun—but you will have to be diligent. A twice-daily application of rich oils or crèmes will need to become second nature, regardless of season.

### Protect

And speaking of sun, the same ideas apply. When it comes to sunscreen, we don't dare leave the house without some kind of SPF on our faces, yet our bodies are often left exposed. The sheer fact that we wear clothes outdoors (well, most of the time) protects areas of the skin from UV damage, but bare limbs in warm weather, and particularly the ultra-vulnerable décolleté and neck areas, require some care. As we age, hyperpigmentation and sun spots can appear seemingly out of nowhere even after just an hour out walking on a sunny day. Of course, we *need* the sun's light, especially by way of the elusive vitamin D—the "sunshine vitamin"—essential for a robust immune system, strong bones, and warding off disease, but we also need it for the sheer mood boost that comes from the solar life-giving force. Vitality is essential to the Witch, and is, quite honestly, mandatory to vibrant beauty. A very effective ritual is to go outdoors, even on a cold day, allowing your body to absorb 10 minutes of pure sunlight. When the season permits, try this in the mornings, before you anoint yourself with beauty potions—maybe step outside with your favorite brew? Expose as much

## BEAUTY WITCH SECRET

*Dry brushing is a fabulous way to get your circulation shimmying while lifting away dull skin. Using a high-quality, eco-friendly brush, begin at your feet and work your way up to your neck with gentle strokes toward the heart (be sure to get in all the little hidden spots, like under your arms and inside your upper thighs.) This ritual is at its most potent during the waning-to-dark moon.*

flesh as the weather allows, invite that delicious fire glow to kiss you, and give thanks. Now you are ready to begin your day from a place of power—don't forget your sunscreen!

## Treat

Just as the face loves masques and treatments, so does the body. Aloe, oatmeal, clay and mud are some of the simplest and most potent full-body treatments that you can easily concoct at home, adding in magickal herbs and oils to suit the lunar cycle and your desires. Spot treatments designed for specific areas are fabulously effective for conditions like acne, dry patches, clogged pores, and irritations, but have you ever experienced a full body masque? It's incredibly sexy. The ritual of covering your entire naked body in texture and scent, then walking around while it works its magick is lusciously *liberating*. As the air hits your potion-cloaked skin, swaying and dancing are most encouraged, followed by a feline stretch before the waterfall of a shower rinses you clean. You emerge feeling divine, in a velvet gown of luminosity … watch out world.

## Spirit Cleanse, Body Wash

Whether you are in need of a boost to greet the new morn, or to chase away energies of the day's passing, this gentle lather will get you balanced. Skin-loving and spirit-lifting, it delicately cleanses the skin without drying, and is suitable for all skin types. This potion is particularly effective before ritual.

### Ingredients

2 oz. rosewater

½ oz. castile soap

2 tablespoons aloe vera extract

13 drops lavender essential oil

8 drops myrtle essential oil

8 drops hyssop essential oil

6 drops rosemary essential oil

**Intention** Purification, balancing, clearing

**Lunar Phase** Waning

**Conjures** 1–2 month supply

## ᐯ Sacred Fire, Body Exfoliant ᐯ

This potion is especially effective for those moments when you need a bit of extra motivation. Monday morning got you down? Dragging yourself through the week? Or perhaps you've lost your drive? Call upon the element of fire to ignite your inner spark.

### Ingredients

½ cup Himalayan pink salt

¼ cup grapeseed oil

1 tablespoon pomegranate powder

8 drops sweet orange essential oil

6 drops frankincense essential oil

**Intention** Motivate, inspire, build momentum, take action

**Lunar Phase** Full

**Conjures** 1–2 treatments

## ᐯ Love Power, Body Exfoliant ᐯ

Draw beauty, love, and abundance to you with this heavenly-scented cauldron of decadence. With this one, you are activating circulation, polishing, and conjuring luminescent radiance. It makes a most satisfying and sensual way to prepare for that other spellbinding ritual: the rendezvous.

### Ingredients

½ cup smoked alderwood salt

¼ cup sunflower oil

Seeds of 1 vanilla bean, scraped

8 drops rose attar

6 drops myrrh essential oil

**Intention** Attraction, love, abundance, glow

**Lunar Phase** New to full

**Conjures** 1–2 treatments

## The Serpent's Secret, Body Exfoliant

In honor of our serpent healers we shed our skin, releasing the old, and letting go of energy which no longer serves us. (Perhaps it never did.) This release is powerful, but protective, as we strip down to prepare for new life. Regeneration is only a potion away.

### Ingredients

½ cup Celtic sea salt

¼ cup sweet almond oil

1 teaspoon horsetail, dried

9 drops juniper essential oil

6 drops lemon essential oil

6 drops geranium essential oil

**Intention** Detoxify, transformation, release, protect

**Lunar Phase** Waning to dark

**Conjures** 1–2 treatments

# Starlight Moonglow, Shimmer Spray Mist

For those enchanted evenings when the only thing to do is to glow like la lune—a softly shimmering blend to cloak your bare skin in pure silver moonlight, with the magick touch of irresistible moisture. Potential suitors beware: your light may simply be too blinding for the faint of heart.

### Ingredients

2 oz. grapeseed oil

1½ oz. sweet almond oil

1 tablespoon rosehip oil

1 tablespoon silver mica powder

1 tablespoon crystal mica powder

**Intention** Shimmer, shine, glow

**Lunar Phase** Waxing to full

**Conjures** 2–3 month supply

# Celestial Body, Moisture Mist

There are few things as sensual as silky, glistening skin. Bare flesh shimmering with moisture and a bit of sheen is wildly sexy to behold, and addictive to touch. Keep this potion close to turn heads and quicken pulses. Should primal urges become unleashed, it is helpful to know that this potion is entirely edible.

### Ingredients

2 oz. grapeseed oil

1 oz. sweet almond oil

½ oz. avocado oil

½ teaspoon vitamin E oil

½ teaspoon vegetable glycerin

Seeds of 1 vanilla bean, scraped

8 drops clove essential oil

**Intention** Moisturize, glow, attract

**Lunar Phase** Waxing

**Conjures** 2–3 month supply

## Children Of the Sun, Body Oil

Though the moon is a magickal super power, it is vital that we also bask in the exuberant radiance of the sun. The life-giving solar force is needed for vitality, energy, and growth, both physically and spiritually—however, we must take care to protect our skin from the dryness inherent with such brilliant light, by anointing it with rich, hydrating moisture, and a light veil of UV protection.

### Ingredients

2 oz. borage seed oil

2 oz. chia seed oil

4 oz. sunflower seed oil

1 tablespoon raspberry seed oil

20 drops carrot seed oil

13 drops sandalwood oil

6 drops jasmine oil

1 small piece of sunstone

**Intention** Deep moisture, sun protection, wrinkle fighting

**Lunar Phase** Waxing to full

**Conjures** 3–4 month supply

## Beauté du Corps Crème, Body Crème

The High Priestess of heavenly body potions. Scented for a celestial courtesan, doused with love and beauty magick, and drenched in moisture that penetrates deeply and locks in hydration, this superior blend caresses your form like the kisses of an ardent lover, with each brush of the lips adding layers of lush sensuality. And then, of course, there is the afterglow…

**Ingredients**
**Phase One**
¼ cup hempseed oil

¼ cup chia seed oil

¼ cup avocado oil

⅓ cup shea butter

**Phase Two**
⅔ cup rosewater

**Phase Three**
20 drops rose attar

1 teaspoon amber resin, crushed to powder

Seeds of one vanilla bean

**Intention** Moisture, hydration, glow, sensuality

**Lunar Phase** Full

**Conjures** 1 month supply

# Temple Pillars, Body Oil

Your lovely legs are the great columns that lead to the inner sanctum of creation. Movement will keep them lean and firm, but the skin isn't always supple. Concoct this potion by the cauldron-full, and use it liberally twice daily to activate circulation, banish toxins, and cast cellulite into the netherworld. An added trick is to employ a magickal tool—the rolling pin—to increase its power by helping to break down fluid retention.

*This potion can also be used on the arms and derriere.

**Ingredients**

2 oz. castor oil

1½ oz. sweet almond oil

1 teaspoon coffee bean extract

20 drops cedarwood essential oil

20 drops geranium essential oil

20 drops rosemary essential oil

10 drops juniper essential oil

8 drops grapefruit essential oil

1 small piece of bloodstone

1 small piece of amber

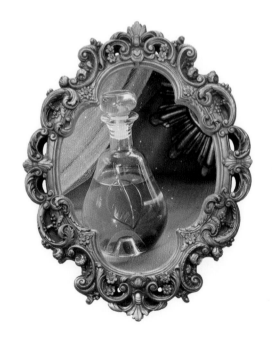

**Intention** Cellulite banishing, circulation boost, firm, detoxify

**Lunar Phase** Waning

**Conjures** 30 treatments

# The Sorceress' Seduction, Body Oil

This intoxicating body nectar makes a beautifying body oil, and a very potent perfume. Apply liberally to channel the one-and-only Inanna—Sumerian sexpot supreme, and Goddess of all things erotic. These magick ingredients literally ooze sex appeal, and light a fire of attraction that draws suitors towards you like moths to the flame. Should you inadvertently drive someone mad with desire, don't say I didn't warn you.

### Ingredients

2 oz. chia seed oil

2 oz. avocado oil

1 teaspoon lapsang souchong tea, dried

8 drops ylang ylang essential oil

6 drops cardamom essential oil

4 drops ginger essential oil

1 piece orange carnelian

1 piece smoky quartz

**Intention** Attraction, sexual prowess, aphrodisiac

**Lunar Phase** Full

**Conjures** 30 treatments

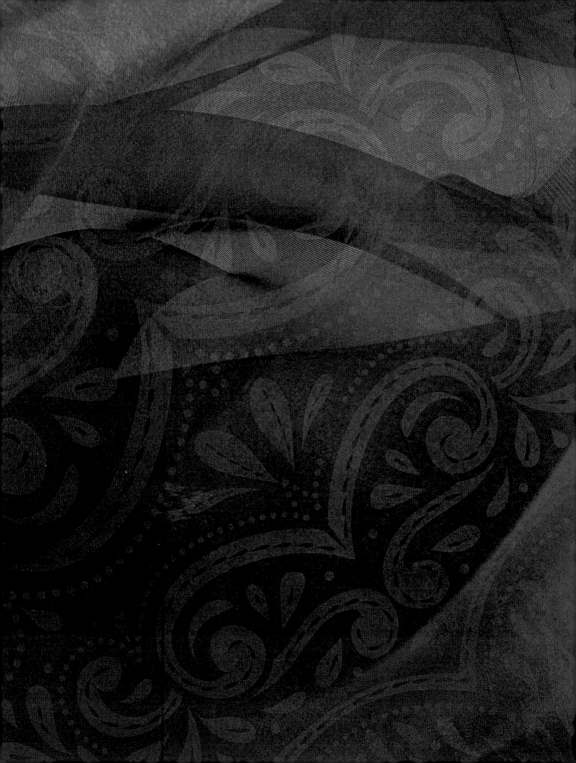

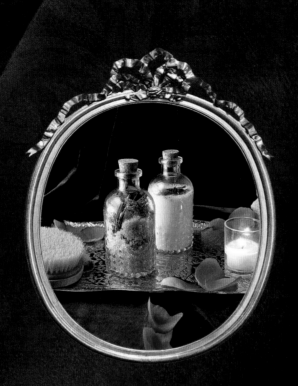

Chapter Twelve

# The Ritual Bath

Oh, to lie back and sink into warm, fragrant waters! To let go of the day and all its cares, closing the door on the rest of the world to a haven of renewal may seem like a luxury that only exists in old movies, but make no mistake: bathing is truly the ultimate ritual for the potent—not to mention glamourous—Witch. It comes alive only in a quiet, candlelit space, where we strip down, piece by piece, the layers of the outer world to enter a scented private ocean of silken waves. The element of water is entirely feminine, representing our ability to create on every level and to nurture those creations throughout their lifetimes. Water heals and purifies, and is vital to all life. It is our emotional body, our intuition, our dreams, and our fluids. The vast oceans that inspire, the mountain streams that flow through the forests, and the raindrops that quench the earth are all symbolic of the very life force that radiates within us: our blood.

As the sacred waters seep into our subconscious via bathing, our intuitive prowess becomes heightened, opening to explore the depths of our innermost selves. From the ocean floor where Yemaya holds court, to the surface where Aphrodite appears, all the mysteries unfold in the timeless expanse between the worlds.

To literally be transformed by surrendering to it seems so oddly out of place in modern life, which is *exactly* what makes it so powerful. Think of it as the classic cinematic bombshell bath that's been touched by a magick wand.

When creating your bathing potions, always add the essential oils and flower essences in one at a time, singing its praises as you hold that visual. If you are making a fresh potion for a single use, pour the salt, base oils, or crèmes into the water first, then add the essential oils. If you wish to store your potion, same thing: add the essentials into the base and stir it well before sealing the vessel.

To make a sachet, simply place your attuned and enchanted herbs (fresh or dried) into a muslin tea bag, or use a small piece of cheesecloth tied with string, and toss the sachet into the running water. Sachets can be made ahead and stored in an airtight glass jar—just be sure to label them.

And, of course, you'll need a beauty cocktail to complete the scene. Sipping a high-vibration libation during your soak heightens the magick *and* the glamour. Concoct a potion from Chapter 16 that suits your mood. And remember that gorgeous vessels are requisite.

# The Ritual of the Bath

### Create Your Sacred Space

As with all of your magickal places, adorn the area with objects which heighten the vibration. For instance, your seaside altar should certainly include at least one candle—

try white for spirit, or yellow for opening up your psychic awareness. Feel free, of course, to add as many as you like to create a heavenly, glamourous environment. You could also add crystals and stones, such as amethyst, moonstone, labradorite and celestite. Foraged, discarded shells are a nice touch, but be aware that larger shells, like conch, are actually shelters for marine life, so be very conscious in your gathering. Beautiful vessels, trays, and bowls are a *must.*

## The World Disappears

This is ritual space, so although it is used practically during other hours, your bath is to be undisturbed by humans, smart phones, and external distractions. (Familiars, naturally, are allowed to barge in at any time they like.) But do invite your favorite water deity as an honored guest—they are always most welcome, and you will find, often the life of the party.

## Gather Your Ritual Needs

Bring all your ingredients in on a beautiful tray or bowl as guided by your intention. Linger for a moment with each one, attuning to their magickal vibration. Include a match or lighter, a candle snuffer, and a fetching robe (with exquisite slippers, of course) to adorn yourself with, après bath.

## Enter the Temple

Close the door, light the candles, and run your bath. As the warm water rises, and steam vapor fills the room, begin to remove your clothing, one piece at a time. Don't rush. With each peel, let go of the world outside. Stresses, concerns, and particularly *thoughts*, are not welcome here—this space is for emotional release, visions, and intuitive communications only. Stretch your limbs and begin to unwind. Run your fingers through your scalp as you gather your hair in a terry wrap to protect it from the steam. When the water is ready, sprinkle each ingredient into this great cauldron before you. Whisper your intention into the gentle waves as they ripple with energy. Swirl the water with your fingertips in symbols appropriate to your intent. Now step in.

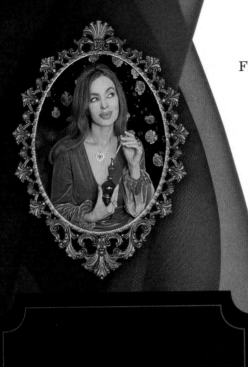

## Float Between the Realms

This is what you've been waiting for. As you submerge into your magickal bath, with heated waters encircling you and fragrance wafting all around, you begin to breathe more slowly. With each inhale, you are drawing your intention closer. With each exhale, you are releasing that which has no business in your sacred space, and ultimately is not needed in your life—anxiety, worry, anger, and fear to name a few—to clear the flow of energy from inside so that your magick can be its most vibrant and effective. Allow yourself to succumb to a trance-like, meditative state as you visualize your wishes, feeling them throughout your body. Send your intentions out into the world, and whisper thanks to the power of water that is aiding you.

## Luxuriate

Now that the work is done, you can play a little. Sip your drink, nibble a strawberry,

### BEAUTY WITCH SECRET

*Sachets can be used in place of essential oils. The scent and healing potency will be stronger with a pure essential oil or flower essence, but the magickal vibration is the same.*

stretch, flip through a vintage magazine … anything that promotes a feeling of glamour, well-being, and a bit of languor.

## Bid it Adieu

Time to rise, my Darlings, just like Aphrodite. Feel the power of your work (and your play) as you emerge, stepping out like a goddess to be contended with. Wrap yourself in a fluffy towel, and as you let the water drain whisper a prayer that any negativity be washed away and rebirthed as healing energy. Now you are ready to anoint your heavenly body with the potions you've created from chapter 13.

# Waning Moon Soak, Bath Salts

This soothing salt potion is a potent purifier that cleanses your physical body and your energetic body, clearing away all negativity and anything which may be clinging to you and weighing you down. It is soothing, detoxifying and calming with an earthy, restorative scent which works best during a waning-to-dark moon, but do reach for it anytime you feel negativity clinging like an ill-fitting dress.

### Ingredients

1½ cups Celtic sea salt

10 drops cedarwood essential oil

8 drops lavender essential oil

8 drops rosemary essential oil

8 drops chamomile essential oil

**Intention** Detoxify, release, clearing

**Lunar Phase** Waning to dark

**Conjures** 1–2 treatments

# Witchy Wellness, Bath Soak

An absolute must for when you are feeling under the weather, this potion soothes body aches, warms chills, lightens a heavy head and helps you to breathe easier. It carries powerful healing magick to nip seasonal suffering in the bud, and also aids in a speedy recovery. You'll be back on your broomstick in no time.

**Sachet**

1 tablespoon, or 2" piece of burdock root

1 tablespoon nettles

**Base**

1 cup Celtic sea salt

1 cup magnesium flakes

1 tablespoon ground mustard seed

**Essential Oils**

10 drops cedarwood

8 drops eucalyptus

8 drops sandalwood

5 drops peppermint

**Intention** Healing, strengthening, soothing

**Lunar Phase** Waxing to full

**Conjures** One treatment

# A Sorceress Prepares, Bath Soak

A ritual bath is a must before more formal magickal workings, and this one is as pleasurable as it is effective. This combination of oils and petals strengthens power to an enviable degree, with the balance of sun and moon aiding your positive intentions to achieve success. Did I mention how divinely sensual it is?

**Sachet**

Petals from three carnation flowers

**Essential Oils**

3 drops ginger

8 drops frankincense

8 drops myrrh

6 drops sandalwood

**Intention** Power, strength, manifestation

**Lunar Phase** Full

**Conjures** One treatment

## Luck Be a Lady, Bath Soak

Though riches come in all forms, who among us couldn't do with a bit more cash? Be it for necessities or a little extra mad money, this blend is concocted to bring treasure to you. And, unlike the song, it's no gamble—pair this bath with unwavering focus, and notice the abundance it draws in.

**Sachet**

3 sticks cinnamon

3 pieces fresh orange peel

1 tablespoon chamomile flowers

**Essential Oils**

10 drops jasmine

8 drops patchouli

**Intention** Money, good fortune, abundance

**Lunar Phase** Full

**Conjures** One treatment

## Cleopatra's Secret, Bath Soak

Egypt's Queen of Seduction bathed her legendary body in milk to keep her skin supple. This luxurious bath crème goes several steps beyond, calling in the nutritive moisturizing powers of coconut and almond for skin that is irresistibly soft, glowing, and somehow entirely ageless. Add in ancient, lusty plant power, and you will exude the magick of timeless allure.

### Sachet

1 teaspoon crushed amber resin

### Base

2 cups coconut milk

2 cups almond milk

### Essential Oils

10 drops myrrh

8 drops neroli

3 drops cinnamon

**Intention** Beauty, youthfulness, sexual prowess, attraction

**Lunar Phase** Full

**Conjures** One treatment

## A Lover's Bath, Bath Soak

Though you have staked your claim on the bathtub as the territory of you and you alone, every so often, it is most enjoyable to share that ritual … with a special someone. Mmm-hmm. Now of course, this is sacred space, so this someone had better be worthy—trust your Witch instincts. Draw this magick bath for the sole purpose of stirring the cauldron of amour, heightening desire, and slowly being fed grapes.

### Sachet
1 cup hibiscus flowers

1 tablespoon damiana

### Base
3 cups almond milk

1 cup rosewater

2 tablespoons vanilla powder

### Essential Oils
12 drops rose absolute

6 drops cardamom

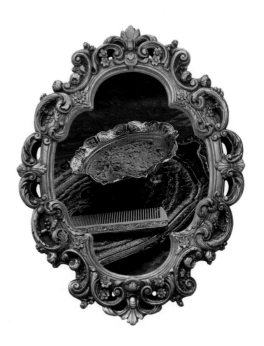

**Intention** Love, romance, sexual desire

**Lunar Phase** New to full

**Conjures** One treatment

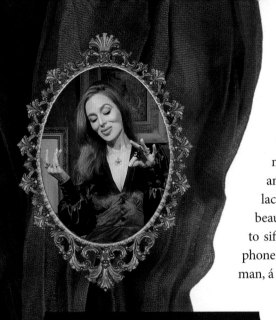

# Bombshell Bubbles, Bath Foam

The ultimate glamour girl soak—up to the neck in effervescent bubbles, hair wrapped in an elegant turban to protect it from the steam, lacquered toes wiggling joyously, candles lit, beauty cocktail in hand, a copy of French vogue to sift through languidly...and a vintage rotary phone at the ready, just in case you need a handyman, á la Marilyn in The Seven Year Itch.

Note: If you have hard water, you may not see much in the way of bubbles. A hard water filter should fix the problem, and is much healthier all around for your skin and hair.

## BEAUTY WITCH SECRET:
### THE TUBBLY

*May I present to you one of my all-time favorite rituals? You guessed it—bubbles in the tub, and bubbles in your glass! Sinking into a bath nearly overfilled with bubbly water, and sipping a good champagne out of a vintage coupe is the cure to anything that could possibly ail you.*

**Ingredients**

1 cup liquid castile soap, unscented

½ cup vegetable glycerin

1 vanilla bean, seeds scraped

13 drops frankincense essential oil

8 drops rose absolute

**Intention** Glamour, beauty, relaxation, enjoyment

**Lunar Phase** Waxing to full

**Conjures** Six treatments

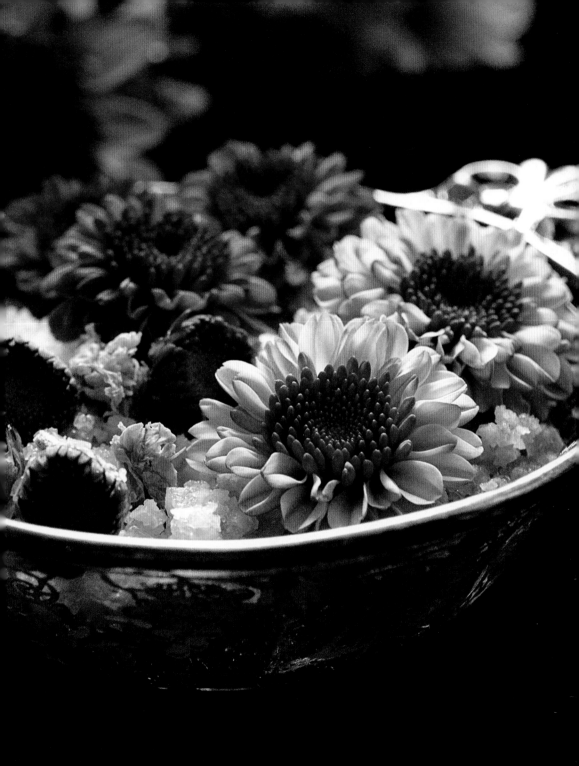

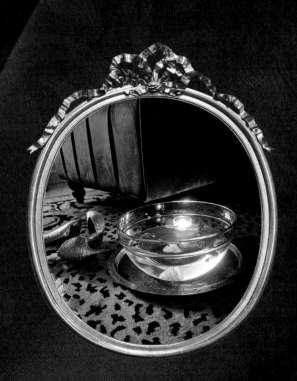

## Chapter Thirteen

# Well Heeled

erhaps the hardest working characters in the cinema of life, feet have the distinction of being employed as unappreciated beasts of burden, required to bear the weight of everyday stress, supporting the entire body (and anything it may be carrying) as they pound the pavement and slush through snow, occasionally finding themselves bathed in mud or submerged in a rain puddle through no fault of their own. Their only real rest comes when we sleep, their only true tending when we treat them to a pedicure. Ironically, our tired tootsies are also the subject of intense, iconic fetishism: from the torturous "lotus foot" binding of Chinese maidens, to the coveted pink satin toe shoe of the prima ballerina, obsessive fixation on the feet cannot be denied.

Then, of course, there is exquisite pain of the high heel, which we gladly succumb to for the sheer love of our most revered accessory. Should a lover dare to sip champagne from a Witches Balenciaga pumps? Never. Her shoes are far too precious.

The naked foot is also a conductor of sensuality, albeit an earthier version. To touch the ground is a communication where spirituality is heightened seemingly without effort. The practice of walking barefoot along the beach, in the grass, or through the forest invites us to connect directly to the energy and electrons of the earth. This ritual immediately boosts our energy and mood, with long term effects of reducing pain and inflammation within the body. A daily promenade along the belly of the mother raises energy—think of tribal dances—as it relieves stress, promotes more restful sleep, and wards off the aging process.

# The Ritual of the Feet

Little treats for your feet are invaluable as a way of relieving muscle stress, cramping, soreness, and casting aside the tension of the day. Put them into practice now, and you will have their benefits for a lifetime. But also do it because it feels ecstatic.

## Stretch

As you wind down your day, one of the nicest things you can do for your feet will also protect them from harm: the oh-so-sensual stretch. Kick off your mules, crouch down on the floor, and place your hands in front of you for support. Now, slowly, rock all the way forward on your toes, giving your arches a languorous stretch. (This feels *so* good, *mes cheris*, you will quickly become hooked!) Hold it all the way forward for a few seconds, then slowly rock all the way back on your heels, hold a moment, then repeat the ritual until your feet are satisfied. They will thank you for decades to come, as this practice wards off foot pain, particularly that which comes from the above mentioned high-heel infatuation.

## Massage

Now here lies a very simple act of ecstasy that can be performed almost anywhere, at any time. Why not kick off your shoes at your desk, on a park bench, or in the locker room of the gym, and give your feet a little love? If you are sporting bare legs, it's especially nice because you can carry a little foot potion in your bag and have a most relaxing, healing little treatment whenever your feet are feeling less than perky. Don't be concerned about anyone seeing you—you are elegantly tending to yourself. Confidently set the example by sitting up straight, gracefully producing a pretty potion bottle from your equally pretty handbag, removing your shoe with sensuality, and gently taking your foot into your hands. The sheer bliss of the experience will give even dubious onlookers pause for thought. They may even ask for your recipe.

## Adorn

Is there anything more cheerful than propping your tired feet upon an ottoman, then glancing down to catch sight of expertly lacquered toes? They wiggle with glee as they show off rich hues and a glossy shine, a reminder that life is, indeed, to be lived. Just as

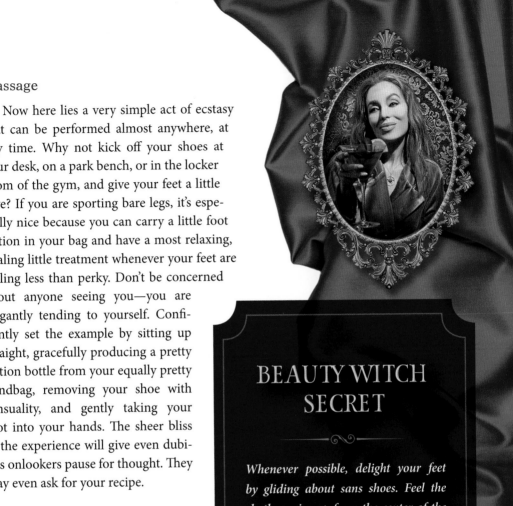

## BEAUTY WITCH SECRET

*Whenever possible, delight your feet by gliding about sans shoes. Feel the rhythms rise up from the center of the earth and up through your soles, all the way out the top of your head, and then back into the cosmos. Indoors or out, the muscles of the feet will become accustomed to your movements, and you will find that whether walking or dancing, the earth will rise to meet you.*

you wouldn't coat your talons with chemically-laden polishes, so should you treat your toes to the same toxin-free polishes out there. Pedicures naturally last longer than manicures (because they don't take the same knocks) so you won't be as tempted to succumb to the gel version if you are heading to the salon—though many now carry a line of natural nail lacquers, too, or mention that you would like to bring your own when booking your appointment. But, of course, the grooming you give yourself in the privacy of your own space can actually be the most fun—the ultimate glamour ritual of the feet includes sipping a glass of bubbly and flipping through a coffee table book while letting your toes dry.

# Well-Heeled Witch, Foot Soak

A gift from the heavens above, and the earth below, for those who worship at the altar of the sky-high heel, this potion is also goddess-sent for anyone who is on their feet all day, even in the sturdiest of cushioned footwear. It reduces swelling, soothes, cools, easing aches and soreness. The epitome of "ahhh" for your tired tootsies, and a blissful evening ritual—even better accompanied by a glass of Bordeaux and a siren's song.

### Ingredients

2 tablespoons St. John's Wort

1 cup spring water

¼ cup Celtic sea salt

¼ cup magnesium flakes

6 drops lavender essential oil

6 drops peppermint essential oil

6 drops tea tree essential oil

**Intention** Healing, soothing, revitalizing

**Lunar Phase** Waning

**Conjures** One treatment

## Kiss the Boot, Foot Crème

For the ultimate mélange of fetish-meets-wellness, whip up this sensual blend for a nightly massage ritual (pun intended.) Infused with eroticism, your feet will be caressed in softness and scent … with the added charm of being entirely edible.

### Ingredients
**Phase One**

⅓ cup cacao butter

¾ cup avocado oil

1 tablespoon candelilla wax

**Phase Two**

⅔ cup rosewater

⅓ cup aloe vera gel

**Phase Three**

1 vanilla bean, seeds only

18 drops cinnamon essential oil

6 drops cardamom essential oil

**Intention** Moisturize, arouse, relieve stress

**Lunar Phase** Waxing to full

**Conjures** 6 month supply

# Tantalizing Toes, Exfoliant & Masque

Polish your feet into a heavenly state of bliss with this brightly scented treatment, designed to revive and rejuvenate. Slough away stale energy, then let it sit a while, allowing the oils and the salt to penetrate. Run your feet under some cool water, and ready yourself for an overwhelming desire to dance.

**Ingredients**

1 cup pink Himalayan salt, finely ground

¼ cup sweet almond oil

¼ teaspoon vitamin E oil

Juice of 1 lemon, or 9 drops lemon essential oil

6 drops lavender essential oil

3 drops rosemary essential oil

**Intention** Cleanse, exfoliate, soften, revive

**Lunar Phase** Waning

**Conjures** 2–3 treatments

# Get On the Good Foot, Foot Masque

There are those less-than glamourous moments when even the most fastidious witch suffers a little foot trouble, by way of an overzealous toenail or a smashing pair of vintage slingbacks that are just a teeny bit too small. Use this super potion to heal ingrowns and any other abrasions with potential for infection. Simply mix all ingredients together, adding spring water a bit at a time, until you have a smooth, fairly thick paste. After cleansing the area gently, apply the mud paste and allow it to sit until it hardens, then rinse with warm water, pat dry, and add a few drops of lavender to protect. Repeat for five days or as needed.

**Ingredients**

2 tablespoons Moroccan red clay

3 drops lavender essential oil

8 drops melaleuca essential oil

6 drops geranium essential oil

4 drops oregano essential oil

1–2 tablespoons spring water, as needed

**Intention** Disinfect, draw out bacteria, healing

**Lunar Phase** Waning

**Conjures** Five treatments

## ⌒ Dancing Days, Foot Mist ⌒

*Mon parole!* A cooling breeze of heaven to kiss your toes, your soles, and even your over-worked calves. Kick up your heels and give them a spritz whenever a lively lift is needed—your co-workers will wonder what's got you giggly.

**Ingredients**

2½ oz. spring water

18 drops peppermint essential oil

8 drops sweet orange essential oil

6 drops clary sage essential oil

**Intention** Cooling, soothing, refreshing

**Lunar Phase** Waxing

**Conjures** 1–2 month supply

# Sweet Stilettoes, Freshening Mist

On occasion, the shadow side of fabulous footwear can arise when you least expect it, and must immediately be banished: the pungent pumps. I know, and I am loathe to even suggest it, but, just in case of emergency, here is a deodorizing potion that really will help. If nothing else, you can liberally spritz your lover's boots—ensuring a harmonious relationship between your couture and their feet, should you happen to share a closet.

**Ingredients**

2 oz. spring water

13 drops geranium essential oil

10 drops lavender essential oil

8 drops eucalyptus essential oil

8 drops wild orange essential oil

**Intention** Freshen, deodorize, scent

**Lunar Phase** Waning

**Conjures** 1–2 month supply

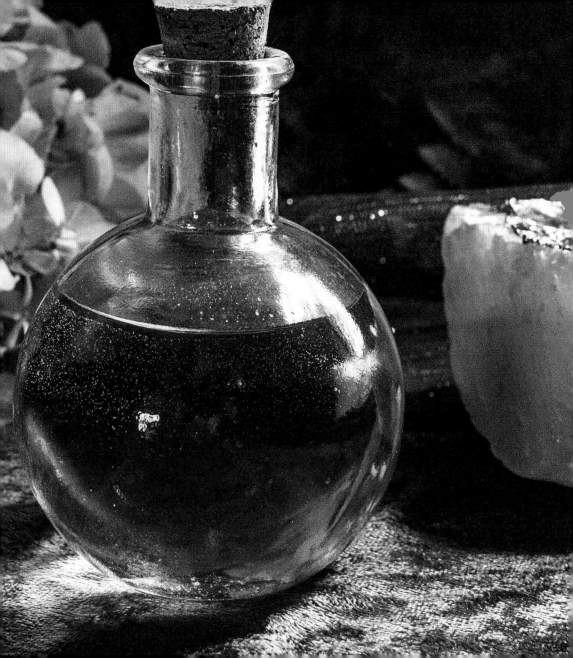

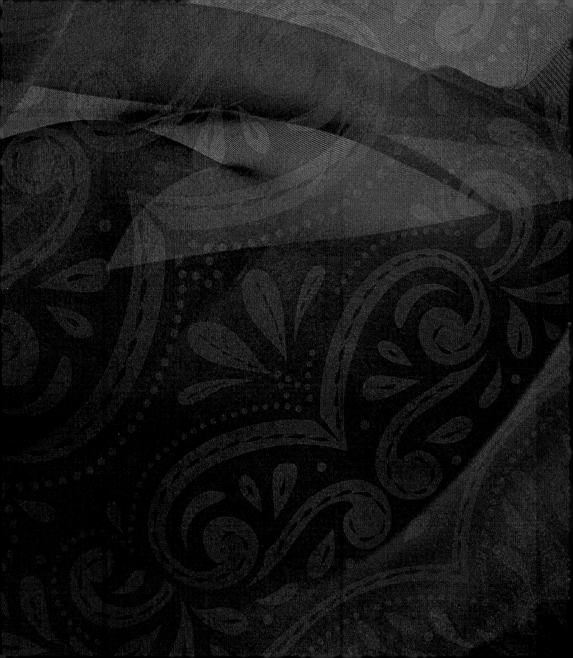

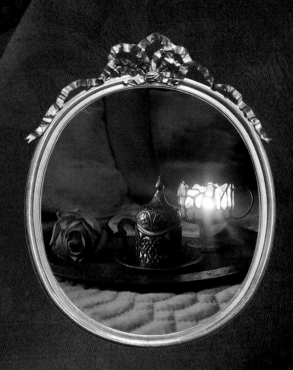

## Chapter Fourteen

# Sleeping Beauty

After the day's adventures turn to the quiet veil of starlight, we begin to create the space for welcoming a most mysterious creature to our inner sanctum: sleep. She is indeed an exalted guest, and so terribly important to us that she usually causes quite a stir. Will she accept our invitation? When will she make her entrance? Will she stay awhile, or just drop in for a moment to be polite? Perhaps she will arrive right on time, speaking softly, with a hostess gift of rest just for us, charmingly wrapped in the silken folds of dreamtime. We love it when she shows up this way. But she is an unpredictable animal, an erratic entry on the guest list we so carefully craft. More often than not, she will decline our request for her stellar presence without so much as an RSVP. (She can be a bit rude.)

We have known this elusive, mysterious femme all our lives. When we were children, she visited often, weaving tales of fantastic journeys and faraway realms into our night flights, opening our consciousness and fine tuning our visions as a foundation for our ever-growing creativity. She then became overpowering in our teens and early twenties, sometimes clobbering us after we'd drank too much, or when we'd pulled a 36-hour study binge. But, as childlike folly dissipates into adult fretting, she finds us less interesting, and begins to show up infrequently to our soirées. By the time we hit our grownup stride, she becomes almost mythological. And, like any great seductress, the harder we pursue her the less interested she is in us.

But what happens when *we* seduce *her*? And how? Subtly, of course, and with total *élan*. You don't lunge at a cat, after all. You go about your business, loving and caring for yourself, and suddenly that indifferent feline wants to sit right in your lap. Now there's sorcery in action.

And, truth be told, as we age we need her more than ever. *Sleep is essential to beauty.* This period of rest allows the body to repair itself by releasing regenerative hormones. When she avoids us, a domino effect of decidedly unappealing events unfold. Lack of sleep literally accelerates the aging process, and not just from the standpoint of what is obvious. We have all met the foes that appear visibly after a restless night, like puffy eyes, dark circles, and dull skin—but what about the damage we can't see immediately? Sleepy heads reach unconsciously for too much caffeine and simple sugars for a boost, resulting in even more fatigue, along with a side of uncomfortable, unflattering bloat. Over time, this leads to dehydration and weight gain. Even worse, sleep deprivation actually speeds aging on all levels by actually *advancing* the process, resulting in brain fog, loss of memory, and depletion of cells.

So, you see, we must cultivate this celebrated creature. You can capture her attention by establishing a nightly ritual that draws such a desirous companion right to you. It isn't difficult, really, but it will require that you change your habits. Out with the televisions and iPads ... make way for the sensuality of slumber!

# The Ritual of Sleep

--•━▶━◀━•--

## The Chamber

Your little cave must be thoughtfully prepared for the ritual of rest. Though it is also your boudoir, adorned for *l'amour*, it must provide the dual function of inviting sleep just as graciously as it does sex. For real REM, we need darkness, we need cool, and we need *quiet*. Invest in heavy draperies, lined in fleece if needed, for optimum blackout. Crack a window, even in winter, whenever possible to circulate fresh air. Use a fan when the air is heavy and stagnant, and treat yourself to a fine mist humidifier when it gets too dry—your skin, hair, and sinuses will thank you. If you have noisy neighbors, try ambient waterfall sounds in the background—it really does work—or conjure a more trancelike temple vibe with sitar music. Set the lights low as you get ready to slip beneath sheets that beckon. Whether you adore crisp cottons or silken petals, keep the quality high and the pillows fluffy. Faerie lights, flameless candles, and salt lamps are a few necessities that will help set the stage for slumber. Aromatherapy in the air and on your linens add another layer of softly pleasurable ambience.

## Release

The body truly readies for rest when tensions are released within the muscles. Make a nightly ritual of stretching your limbs and getting the kinks out, then slipping into a soothing bath. Soaking away aches while clearing your mind work wonders for letting go of what can prevent sleep from showing up. Even a quick shower is helpful, acting as both a body soother and spirit-cleansing waterfall.

## Sip

Part of your evening ritual may need to include a petite brew designed for relaxation and sleep. It's best to drink a potion at least an hour or two before you wish to drift off,

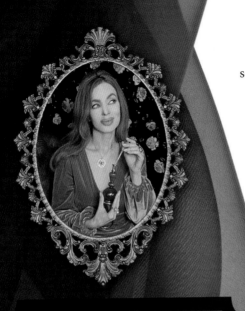

so pesky powder room visits don't wake you later on. With each sip, warm, restful brews signal the brain and body to still, allowing the benefits of plant power to really work while you go about your evening ritual.

### Breathe

And, at last, as you sink into this heavenly down of comfort, you must clear the mind of any lingering chattiness. Meditations for sleep are *so* potent here—if you haven't tried them, do. If something is troubling you, journal it out of the brain and onto the page, then close the book. Slow your breathing to a rhythmic calm, close your eyes, and feel yourself reclining in your ultimate nest: upon a wave of stars, in a bed of flowers, or nestled close to your power animal atop velvety moss. Play a little, and find what gives you that final *"ahhh"* before drifting off.

## BEAUTY WITCH SECRET

*The three nights of the full moon are notorious for disrupting beauty sleep. But don't get upset—this is a Witches power time. If you are kept awake, use the silent hours to bask in the silver light, either through a window or outdoors. Be open to the information coming in. Listen. Feel. Use it.*

# Perchance to Dream, Body & Aura Mist

A light spritz of this calming, restful mist from head to toe will ready your senses for slumber. Like faerie dust, it cloaks you in its magick, with the added benefits of dewy moisture and delicious aromatherapy.

**Ingredients**

2½ oz. spring water

1 teaspoon passion flower, dried

1 teaspoon chamomile, dried

13 drops lavender essential oil

20 drops yarrow essential oil

**Intention** Stress relief, relaxation, peace, sleep, protection

**Lunar Phase** Waning to dark

**Conjures** 1–2 month supply

# You Are Getting Sleepy, Brew

Truly a Witches brew, this contains the strongly scented and slightly bitter valerian root, a powerful magick herb for inducing sleep. As you sip it, you feel immensely relaxed, almost as if entered into an altered and elevated state. But not to worry, you are watched over. Your bliss becomes beauty rest that will leave you feeling refreshed and clear when you wake.

Note: Take caution not to drive after sipping, and do not mix with alcohol or other sedatives.

**Ingredients**

1 cup dark moon water, or pure spring water

1 teaspoon valerian root, dried

½ teaspoon lavender, dried

1 teaspoon stevia, or to taste

**Intention** Relax, induce restful sleep, protect

**Lunar Phase** Dark

**Conjures** 1 serving

## Between the Worlds, Linen Mist

Now that you've sipped, stretched, and misted, you are ready to slip between the sheets for a blissful rest. What could possibly make your slumber more magickal? Deliciously scented linens. Aromatic waves of dreamy delight surround you with their sorcery—you may just be seduced into going to bed a bit earlier!

**Ingredients**

3 oz. spring water

10 drops cedarwood essential oil

8 drops marjoram essential oil

8 drops chamomile essential oil

Seeds of ½ vanilla bean, scraped

**Intention** Calm, aid relaxation, healing, protection, sleep

**Lunar Phase** Dark

**Conjures** 1–2 month supply

# Goodnight Kiss, Sleep Balm

Oh, just one last kiss … but this one you can give to yourself. Massage a small amount of this heavenly balm into your temples to clear your thoughts, soothe your mind, and lighten your entire being before drifting off. It even does wonders for a slight headache. Perhaps you will awaken to an altogether different kind of kiss—the kind that will keep you in bed. Sweet dreams.

**Ingredients**

**Phase One**

1 oz. avocado oil

1 oz. rosehip oil

1 oz. candelilla wax

**Phase Three**

20 drops chamomile essential oil

13 drops peppermint essential oil

13 drops lavender essential oil

8 drops rosemary essential oil

**Intention** Calm, soothe, relieve pressure, sleep, protect

**Lunar Phase** Waning to dark

**Conjures** 2–3 month supply

## BEAUTY WITCH SECRET

*Burning pure valerian incense in your sleep chamber before bedtime will create a relaxed, slightly woozy vibration in the room, aiding your rest. Be sure to snuff it out completely before you close your eyes, bien sûr.*

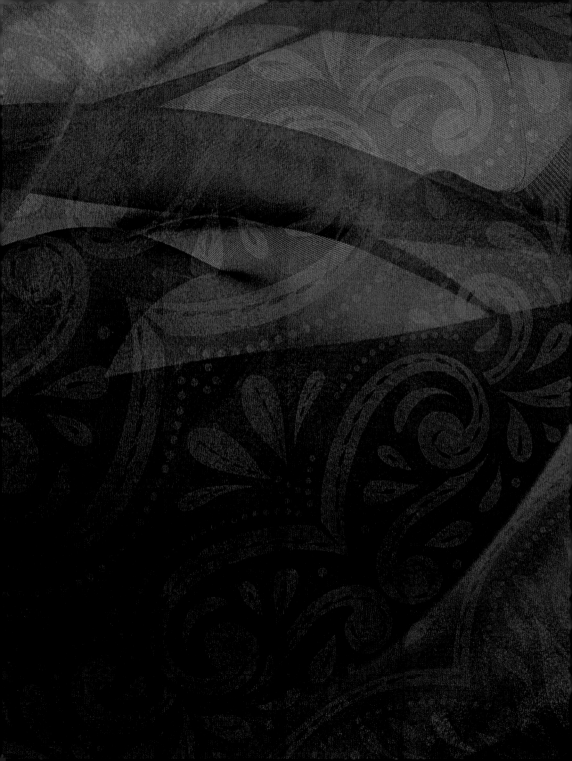

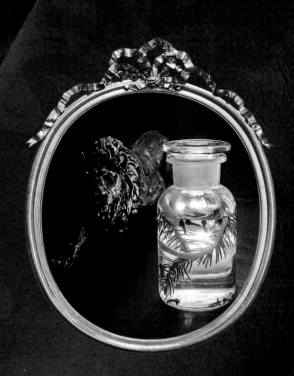

Chapter Fifteen

# For the Wizards in Your World

𝒜h, men. Just as traditional witchcraft celebrates both God and Goddess as a union of divine power and balance—as Lord and Lady of the Forest, Sun and Moon, sky and sea, fire and water, earth and air—so we honor the gentlemen rogues and wise wizards in our lives. And why shouldn't we? Men need sexy grooming rituals too, along with effective potions that are free of chemicals. Of course, the fellas are most welcome to try any of the potions in this book, and indeed will benefit from them, with the exception of those specific to women's health. But if they themselves aren't particularly Witch-crafty, treat your cherished lover, father, brother, or friend to these spell-binding blends, conjured with adoration and sprinkled with the healing magick of the sorceress.

# The Wizard, Beard Oil

Have you ever met a wizard without a lustrous beard? You never will. Impressive facial hair is as much the trademark of the sage as is the staff (which we will get to later, ahem.) Whether he appears as the archetypal sorcerer of old with a long, lush goat's growth or as a modern magus with more refined whiskers, his needs will be the same: keep it soft, and avoid ingrown hairs and other facial eruptions at all costs. This potion does it all with a fetching forest scent that's sure to entice. One teaspoon of castor oil can be added if length is being encouraged, or if he desires to fill in a few sparse areas. Massage a small amount into beard (and the skin beneath) twice daily for maximum potency.

**Ingredients**

1 oz. hemp seed oil

1 oz. jojoba oil

½ oz. brahmi oil

8 drops cedar wood essential oil

6 drops clove essential oil

6 drops pine essential oil

**Intention** Moisturized, smooth, soft, clear pores

**Lunar Phase** New to full

**Conjures** 2–3 month supply

# The Warrior's Sword, Shave Crème

For the wizard who wants to banish those errant hairs that threaten the sheer magnificence of his bristles by growing where he wishes they wouldn't. Also a welcome friend to that knight in shining armor you may know who must sometimes appear incognito—as a clean-shaven modern man about town. Follow directions for making crèmes (p. 48–50), but note that this recipe does not contain rosewater—the aloe vera will heat quickly as it is a small amount. Chill the finished mixture overnight before blending for a fluffy texture. Ladies, this is also fabulous for you!

**Ingredients**

**Phase One**

¾ cup shea butter

½ cup coconut oil

3 tablespoons sweet almond oil

**Phase Two**

2 tablespoons aloe vera gel

**Phase Three**

1 tablespoon baking soda

8 drops lavender essential oil

8 drops sandalwood essential oil

**Intention** Softening, protecting, clarifying

**Lunar Phase** Waning

**Conjures** 2–3 month supply

## A Splash of Sorcery, After Shave

After that expert exorcism of unwanted bristles, he needs cooling. Free of alcohol, this potion soothes and disinfects post-shave skin with a gentle caress, cloaking him in the scent of a rather dapper pirate. Simply combine all ingredients, mix well, then decant into a dashing spray or cologne bottle, as is the gentleman's preference.

### Ingredients

2 oz. liquid aloe vera

2 tablespoons sweet almond oil

3 tablespoons spring water

1 tablespoon cucumber extract

10 drops chamomile essential oil

10 drops calendula essential oil

8 drops bay laurel essential oil

*Note: Shake well before each use, as contents settle.*

**Intention** Calm, refreshed, protected

**Lunar Phase** New to waxing

**Conjures** 1–2 month supply

## Essence de l'homme, Cologne

Whatever his role in your life, the wizard who receives this gorgeous gift will thank you for the spell it casts upon his lover. An irresistible cauldron of scent, at once both gallant and refined, will invite his *amoureuse* (or *amoureux*, as the case may be) ever-close, and keep that special someone coming back for more. How luscious if it happens to be you!

### Ingredients

2 oz. spring water

18 drops sandalwood essential oil

16 drops frankincense essential oil

10 drops cedarwood essential oil

8 drops clove essential oil

8 drops fir essential oil

6 drops lemon essential oil

*Note: Shake well before each use, as contents settle.*

**Intention** Allure, confidence, sensuality

**Lunar Phase** New to full

**Conjures** 1–2 month supply

## Conjuring Follicles, Hair Treatment

Often the mature magus needs a little bit of hocus pocus to feather his cap, so to speak. A regular ritual of applying this potion will do just that—it contains powerful ingredients to boost circulation to the scalp, assist in new healthy growth, and raise a protective shield against the hormone (DHT) that causes hair loss. Feel free to adjust the essential oils to heighten the scent to his liking. This is best concocted in a bowl first before decanting into a glass jar. A quarter-sized dollop is massaged into the scalp, and allowed to rest for at least ten minutes (but it can sit for hours if you have time,) then washed with a gentle shampoo. Better yet, do it for him.

### Ingredients

1 oz. pumpkin seed oil

1 oz. black cumin seed oil

2 tablespoons brahmi oil

1 tablespoon castor oil

10 drops clary sage essential oil

8 drops cedarwood essential oil

8 drops rosemary essential oil

**Intention** Growth, protection, circulation

**Lunar Phase** Full

**Conjures** Twelve treatments

# The Horned God, Elixir

As the consort of the Goddess, he is the male half of the spiritual union: the horned lord of the forest—wild, fertile, earthy—the hunter and the hunted, the sun to her moon. Half man, half beast, he conjures the most primal creative force within the male. After all, the Wizard's staff (ahem)is how he conducts energy. Guide him back to his inner Horned God with this spirited shake, fortified with pure power and guaranteed to awaken his libido. Add the tea to the elixir ingredients and blend well. Then get ready…

## Ingredients

### Tea

1 teaspoon horny goat weed

1 teaspoon saw palmetto berries

1 cup spring water

### Elixir

1 cup mango, cubed, fresh or frozen

1 large carrot, or two smaller ones

½ teaspoon maca powder

1 teaspoon ashwagandha powder

1 teaspoon pine pollen

3 dates, pitted and chopped

Seeds of one vanilla bean, or 1 teaspoon vanilla powder

½ cup unsweetened almond milk

**Intention** Sex drive, virility, energy

**Lunar Phase** Full

**Conjures** One serving

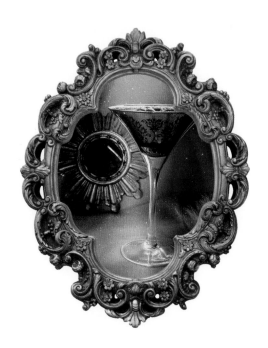

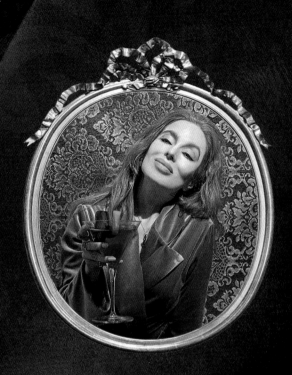

## Chapter Sixteen

# Witches Brews

*J*ust as the cauldron betokens abundance, so does the chalice—the vessel of female creation placed upon the altar, used in ceremony, and indeed represented in the practical magick of sipping a beauty cocktail. As beauty begins on the inside, high-vibration libations become a cornerstone of daily ritual—a bespoke menu of tonics conjured to suit your every need. A well-crafted drink enhances beauty while drawing magickal benefits to she who sips it.

Consider the idea of "drinking your powers." What if every beverage that touched your lips contained spellbinding secrets? When you make the choice to feed your beauty, you also fortify your strength, your intellect, your *potency*. This makes you a force to be reckoned with. Whereas ordinary sips can actually deplete your beauty, "Craft cocktails" enhance every inch of you. Truly powerful Witches are *healthy*. Your magick depends on your strength, wellness, and balance, so keeping yourself in tip top form is actually one of the most important things you can strive for. Detoxing, fueling, and hydrating with beauty beverages is an easy way to ingest plant magick. And it's deeply pleasurable.

Now, of course, it is nearly impossible to omit coffee and champagne from our lives altogether—and why would we ever want to? The objective here is not to obliterate fun, but rather *add* to it. When we expand our repertoire of beverages to include those that infuse us with life force, we open up to endless possibilities. There are myriad ways to incorporate petite upgrades throughout your day and night that bequeath enormous benefits. The conscious act of preparing with magickal intent elevates the potion to even higher levels. Why not, from time to time, replace that first cup with a morning cauldron mug of Focus Pocus (p. 188–189)? Something to get you moving that *also* brightens your complexion is far superior to a sip that dehydrates, triggers stress hormones, and causes bloating, no? And, instead of an "energy" drink in the afternoon, what if you enjoyed an elixir or brew that not only gave you the boost you needed to get through the rest of the day, but also plumped your skin? And how about raising the bar on social and celebratory drinking? The idea of infusing your evening cocktail with super powers is just downright sexy.

Though it never actually happened this way historically, the legend is fun, so go with me here: If Dom Pérignon likened his first heady experience of bubbly to that of "drinking stars" imagine, on a magickal level, if you committed to drinking in cosmic consciousness *every single day*. It's entirely transformational. And yet another way to empower yourself.

# Elixirs

When a power surge is required to feed your hungry spirit and revive your heavenly body to its fullest, reach for a silky, satisfying elixir. Always abundant with comely nutrients, these beauty blends feed you on every level. Think of them as a glamorous, enchanted alternative to the ubiquitous, awkwardly-dubbed "smoothie."

## Green Beauty

All hail *La Déesse du Matin*! She is the High Priestess of the New Day, abundant with the powers of bright energy and a dazzling lust for life. Sip this slowly while preparing for your daily adventures, easing your body into receiving nutrition as you absorb the pure vitality of its magick—your skin, eyes, and whole being will glow! Feel free to mix it up seasonally, just keep the greens-to-fruit ratio heavy on the leafy side, adding cooling or warming spices as the temperatures feed your desires.

Note: This can be made the night before and stored in the refrigerator to make it easy in the morning—just give it a good shake before drinking. And do add a banana and a tablespoon of chia seeds, if you like, for a more robust meal with a kiss of protein.

### Ingredients

1 cup spinach

1 cup kale, stems removed

½ sweet apple, such as Pink Lady or Gala

½ inch piece ginger root, peel removed

1 teaspoon dried nettles

½ teaspoon matcha powder

¼ cup unsweetened almond milk, or ½ teaspoon unrefined coconut oil

¾ cup spring water

Juice of 1 lemon

1 teaspoon cinnamon

1–2 packets of stevia, as desired

**Intention** Rev circulation & digestion, energize, feed

**Lunar Phase** New

**Conjures** One serving

## The Bunny Shake

For the love of vintage men's magazines and all the naturally beautiful ladies that graced their pages. For a time when bodies were goddess-given, and faces were unique. For all the Bunnies dolled up in candy-colored satins, with big lashes and hair, looking like glamour on fire.

This is my offering: Spicy-sweet, colorful, and brimming with beauty prowess—a toast to the golden era of style.

**Ingredients**

3 carrots, finely chopped, or 1 cup unsweetened carrot juice

¾ cup unsweetened almond milk

1 teaspoon garam masala

1 teaspoon cinnamon

1 pinch cloves

Seeds of 1 vanilla bean, scraped

Stevia to taste

**Intention** Increase metabolism, boost immunity, heals skin, hydrates

**Lunar Phase** Waxing

**Conjures** One serving

## The Cacao God

There are sexier rituals than consuming chocolate, yes, but most everything can be beautifully enhanced by a taste of the deep dark stuff. Fiery and virile, cacao is a potent male energy once used as currency, drank in ritual, and later consumed in secret as a forbidden aphrodisiac. It is the Cacao God's offering to the Feminine Divine—and divine it is. Naturally she accepts with her signature aplomb. Fill yourself with its life force whenever you need an extra push of strength and power, both mental and physical.

### Ingredients

1 cup unsweetened cashew milk

1 tablespoon raw, unsweetened cacao powder

2 tablespoons black chia seeds

¾ cup dates, pitted and chopped

1 tablespoon raw hemp seeds

1 teaspoon ashwagandha powder

½ teaspoon ground cinnamon

¼ teaspoon ground cardamom

**Intention** High energy, mental clarity, strength, beautifying

**Lunar Phase** Full

**Conjures** One serving

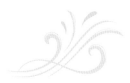

# Spirit Guide

For those moments when you need to be at your strongest, inside and out. A tropical alternative to our delightful chocolate blend, this potion fortifies and energizes with the aphrodesia of sweet fruit nectar in a deeply beautifying drink to satisfy the body's needs. To make the chia seed gel, simply whisk three tablespoons of chia seeds with 1 cup of spring water, then let it set 30 minutes to allow the seed to absorb the water, creating a "gel." Whisk it several times while it sits to avoid clumps, and chill the leftovers for tomorrow's elixir!

**Ingredients**

1 cup unsweetened cashew milk

1 banana

1 cup frozen mango

¼ cup chia seed gel

1 teaspoon ground cinnamon

1 teaspoon raw coconut nectar

pinch saffron threads

**Intention** Strengthen, energize, build collagen, hydrate, firming

**Lunar Phase** Full

**Conjures** One serving

# Voluptuous Vixen

Here is the Witch at her most female, sensual, mythical. Not feeling it at the moment? You will be. The ritual of concocting this potion followed by the unparalleled pleasure of sipping it will get you there. Rich and creamy, it exemplifies la femme in all her fullness—a cornucopia of beauty, love, and desire.

**Ingredients**

½ cup strawberries

½ avocado

¾ cup plain unsweetened coconut yogurt

½ cup unsweetened coconut milk

2 tablespoons raw coconut nectar

Seeds of 1 vanilla bean, scraped

1 tablespoon organic rose water

**Intention** Hydrate, plump and firm skin, smooth lines, radiance

**Lunar Phase** Full

**Conjures** One serving

## Nectar of the Goddess

Who says a cleanse has to be boring? I have something much more fun in mind: an elixir that drenches you in luxurious ambrosia, giving pure pleasure as it keeps your body and skin clear. For your added enjoyment, age-defying magick is at work here, a reminder that nature has you covered.

**Ingredients**

1 cup unsweetened cashew milk

2 nectarines, chopped

1 cup white seedless grapes

⅛ teaspoon ground cinnamon

1 teaspoon stevia or coconut nectar, or to taste

**Intention** Cleanse, anti-aging, hydrate

**Lunar Phase** New

**Conjures** One serving

## Lavender Love Child

Another delight for oily or combination skin, this time nestled in a flower field amongst juicy berries. Go there, strip down, and lose yourself in the lusciousness of the moment knowing that you grow more gorgeous with each sip.

### Ingredients

1 cup unsweetened almond milk

1 banana, frozen

1 cup fresh blueberries

1 tsp dried lavender

1 lemon, zested and juiced

1 teaspoon stevia, or to taste

**Intention** Purify, firm, fight wrinkles

**Lunar Phase** New

**Conjures** One serving

## Ruby Slippers

When stress hits, you lose sight of your own well-being, and it manifests directly on your face. Irritations, dryness, and breakouts—not to mention a bloaty belly—suddenly appear, making things infinitely worse. No need to click your heels, though. Conjure this potion and be transported to a magickal place where everything you need to rejuvenate is in one delectable drink. Deeply detoxing, age-defying, and replenishing with potent red fruits that support your root chakra, it is a much-needed breath of fresh air for your entire being.

### Ingredients

1 cup unsweetened almond milk

1 cup cranberries

1 small beet root

1 tablespoon raw coconut nectar

1 sprig fresh mint

Pomegranate seeds for garnish

**Intention** Detoxifying, cleansing, age-defying, rejuvenating

**Lunar Phase** Waning

**Conjures** One serving

## ◌— The Royal Purple —◌

Inspired by the Byzantine empress Theodora, this potion bears her powers as a stage actress, famous courtesan, and regal advocate for women's rights. One tough cookie, she suffered no fools, and would prefer that you didn't either. Consume this in the unwavering spirit of strength, determination, and tenacity while holding space for her legendary beauty and wit. (Just leave out the bit about her being ruthless—take the high road instead.)

### Ingredients

1 cup unsweetened cashew milk

1 plum, chopped

½ cup fresh blackberries

½ cup goji berries, plus a few for garnish

¼ small avocado

1–2 tablespoons maple syrup, to taste

**Intention** Build collagen, fight wrinkles, promote elasticity, strengthen

**Lunar Phase** Full

**Conjures** One serving

# Brews

Oh, to stir the cauldron over a fire as the fragrant mist tickles your nose (and opens your pores!) A richly prepared brew fortifies, empowers, and returns us to the earth every time; back to our "roots," so to speak! Though these are usually served hot, they can, of course, be enjoyed iced when a cool infusion of beauty sorcery beckons.

## Focus Pocus

I would never dream of depriving you of a hot cup of something fabulous in the morning. I will however, in a heartbeat, suggest cutting back a bit on your consumption of le café. Coffee, delightful as it is, dehydrates the entire body—this translates to a tired-looking face and tummy issues, along with the inevitable crash. Try this brew instead, or at least intermittently, to give your beauty a break. It makes the ideal 4-cup French press for chic serving, sharing, and staying hot. Speaking of hot, have you seen yourself since making this part of your morning ritual?

### Ingredients
1 teaspoon loose chai tea blend

1 teaspoon Lion's Mane mushroom powder

1 teaspoon snow lotus mushroom powder

1 teaspoon raw cacao powder

4 cups spring water

stevia and nut or seed milk to taste

**Intention** Energize, fortify, strengthen, mental clarity, hydration, beautifying

**Lunar Phase** Waxing to full

**Conjures** 4 servings

## Bitches Brew

Oh, the joys of navigating your own lunar cycle. Fortunately, you have back up: this take-no-prisoners blend overpowers cramps, mood swings, bloating and general stress with pure Witch power. It also softens your edgy outlook—it's gorgeous to inhale, to sip, and to be near. Concoct a cauldron full to have on hand when monthly malaise inevitably strikes.

**Ingredients**

1 teaspoon chamomile

3 star anise seeds, crushed slightly

6 juniper berries

½ teaspoon fennel seed

½ teaspoon skullcap, dried

½ teaspoon coriander seeds, crushed slightly

½ teaspoon cinnamon, powdered

½ teaspoon white willow bark

¼ teaspoon cumin seed

seeds of ½ vanilla bean

2 cups spring water

**Intention** Relieve pain, ease stress, mood lifting, release excess fluids

**Lunar Phase** Waning

**Conjures** Two servings

## The Lady Fair

Mundane afternoon sips are for ordinary creatures. Elevate your daytime drinks to bombshell status by brewing the ultimate beauty potion instead, to enjoy hot or iced, all year long. Infused with hydration, vitamins, and antioxidants for all-day radiance, this packs a serious beauty punch, cumulative and enviable, while instilling a bright and gracious energy. Watch their expressions as you age backwards.

### Ingredients

1 teaspoon rosehips

1 teaspoon rose petals

1 teaspoon hibiscus flowers

1 teaspoon calendula flowers

1 teaspoon schisandra berry

1 teaspoon white peony root

½ teaspoon snow lotus mushroom powder

2 cups spring water

**Intention** Hydration, youthful skin, energy, calm

**Lunar Phase** Waxing to full

**Conjures** Two servings

## Wild Things

When life is in overdrive, everything is spinning, and your brain refuses to be quiet, you need a dose of wild magick. Inspired by Diana, Ancient Lady of the Beasts, this potion does the trick. When stress hits hard, cortisol skyrockets—signaling the body to accelerate the aging process. This is not acceptable. Call upon the Mistress of Wild Things for the restoration of your feral self, casting a spell of inner peace to help you listen to the rhythm of nature instead of those silly voices that invade your head.

### Ingredients

1 teaspoon licorice root

1 teaspoon cats claw, dried

1 teaspoon pau d'arco, dried

1 cinnamon stick

1 lemon wedge

1 cup spring water

Stevia to taste

**Intention** Relieve stress & adrenal fatigue, calm, restore

**Lunar Phase** Waning

**Conjures** One serving

# Rich Witch

Rather than waiting for a market crash before working some money magick, why not draw abundance to you all the time? Call upon the Queen of Pentacles as you sip this potion in your ritual bath (see Luck Be a Lady, p. 147–148) as you bring riches near. As always, beautifying plant power is present for supreme confidence and good health, which you will need to enjoy all that cash coming in.

**Ingredients**

1 teaspoon pineapple powder

Peel of ½ orange

2 mint leaves

¼ inch piece ginger root, peeled

1 cup spring water

Stevia to taste

**Intention** Rev circulation, strengthen, boost immunity, increase collagen production

**Lunar Phase** Waxing

**Conjures** One serving

# A Sip of Sorcery

The ideal companion to your ritual bath (see A Sorceress Prepares, p. 146–147), this warm brew prepares you for magick-making. Enjoy its earthy, slightly sweet body entwined with celestial vibes as you feel your power rising, your focus streamlined, and the gentle release of distracting energy.

**Ingredients**

3 star anise, crushed slightly

1 sprig rosemary, or ½ teaspoon dried

½ teaspoon lavender flowers

1 cup spring water

Coconut milk and stevia to taste

**Intention** Cleanse, prepare, focus

**Lunar Phase** Dark to new

**Conjures** One serving

## 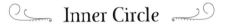 Inner Circle

No matter where you are, a protective circle can be conjured. Your mind's eye is your most powerful tool, but it can be aided and abetted by this bit of potion witchery: an enduring blend of protective plants to cast an energetic shield wall around you. You will find this particularly effective at work—try placing a large vessel-full right next to you at your desk. Its presence alone will warn those who are toxic to stay at a respectful distance. I recommend an unblinking stare to accompany this gesture.

### Ingredients

¼" burdock root

1 teaspoon mugwort, dried

1 teaspoon rose petals

1 teaspoon violet flowers (dried violet leaf will work well also)

1 cup spring water

Stevia to taste

**Intention** Ward off illness, protect, beautify, strengthen

**Lunar Phase** Full

**Conjures** One serving

# Beauty Cocktails

———•▸•◂•———

Sultry, celebratory cocktails are not only mandatory in the life of a sexy Witch, they are the cherries on top of a successful week. This does not mean they have to contain spirits, of course, that part is entirely up to you. Each potion conjured here has been crafted with your beauty in mind, in particular the hydration needed to balance the drying effects of alcohol, and they are delightful on their own if you prefer them virgin. In fact, beauty beverages like kombucha, teas, and plant-derived waters make excellent substitutes for their boozy counterparts—try them! Of course, if you like a kick, the spirits here do contain some positive benefits, so be sure to look them up in the Ingredients index (p. 203). As a general rule, blend all nonalcoholic ingredients together, fill your chalice ¾ full, then add a robust splash of "poison"—if you prefer to measure, approximately ¼ cup of booze. This gives each drink some life without letting you get too far gone. A magickal glass of water before and after salutations will be most welcomed by your body, too, as it will help soften the effects of indulging. *À votre santé!*

## The Pink Panther

Slink around your Lair like the most glamorous feline that ever prowled in the moonlight, cocktail glass in hand, filled to its delicate rim with bombshell beauty. This one is playful, coy, and beyond sexy. Try it with a splash of bubbly for big-cat effervescence—the night is young, and so is your skin. Meow!

**Ingredients**

1 cup cactus water

1 small watermelon

1 cup raspberries

2 large mint leaves

½ teaspoon catnip

3 drops lime essential oil

Champagne

**Intention** Hydrate, defy aging, strengthens skin, boost immune system

**Lunar Phase** Waxing

**Conjures** One serving

## The Cosmo Girl

The vintage Cosmo Girl had it all: a chic apartment, dazzling career, fabulous friends, and a sizzling love life—with the purrfect wardrobe to suit every occasion. Everywhere she went, she brought style, smarts, and sex appeal. Step into her expert heels and be inspired to have exactly the life you wish for, with a little help from your magickal friends. Allow the hibiscus flowers and rosehips to steep in the spring water for 30 minutes ahead, and break out the martini glasses for this one! This recipe makes a carafe-full to have on hand the next time you host a fête for the fantastic females that orbit around you.

### Ingredients

8 cups spring water

3 tablespoons hibiscus flowers

2 tablespoons rose hips

3 drops lemon essential oil

Splash of pomegranate juice

Orange slices to garnish

Fine pink Himalayan salt for rim

Gin

**Intention** Hydrate, fight wrinkles, firm, nourish

**Lunar Phase** Waxing to full

**Conjures** 8-cup carafe

# Strawberry Starlight

The purrfect Mars-Venus alignment! A lusty connection is made beneath the night sky for your pleasure, and that special consort you share it with. Though we always associate wine with Bacchus, the earliest wine deities were actually female: in ancient Mesopotamia, twelve vases per day were offered to Ishtar! White wine is lunar-ruled, so be sure to sip beneath her luminescent light.

### Ingredients
5 large basil leaves

¾ cup spring water

3 strawberries

Dry white wine, such as a sauvignon blanc

Basil for garnish

**Intention** Age-defying, protective, collagen-boosting, hydrating

**Lunar Phase** Waxing

**Conjures** One serving

# ❧ Orange Skies ❧

Oooh! This one is frisky! The citrus fruits here are a beautiful balance of solar and lunar energies, so this makes a lovely afternoon libation as well as an evening cocktail. With a whirl of kaleidoscopic dreams, it bestows sexual freedom and pure love. Lose yourself in it.

### Ingredients

6 mint leaves

1 cup spring water

½ orange, seeded and cut into wedges

Juice of two lemon wedges

Gin

**Intention** Boost immune system, sensuality, hydrate, brighten

**Lunar Phase** Waxing

**Conjures** One serving

# ❧ Moonlight Margaritas ❧

Oh yes. We are going there. With a bombshell's twist of ingredients, the classic midnight conga-line-and-fortune-telling party becomes beautified with skin-loving hydration, vitamins, and minerals to balance the spirits, both in your glass and those hovering about. Pop all the ingredients into a blender, then pour into a salt-rimmed goblet, garnish, and let loose. Just keep a close eye on that rose garden—has it grown wildly overnight?

### Ingredients

2 cups coconut water

12 ice cubes

2 cups frozen pineapple

Juice of 2 limes, plus several for garnish

2 teaspoons coconut nectar

Celtic salt, finely ground

Tequila

**Intention** Hydration, repair skin damage, fight wrinkles

**Lunar Phase** Full

**Conjures** Four servings

## The Bond Girl

Wherever would 007 be without all those drop-dead dames? My guess is retired long ago. This bewitched variation of the iconic Vesper packs as much punch as its namesake, but this time with the lady in mind: beautifying, clever, and protective to keep your heavenly body happy, inside and out. Let the juniper berries steep in the water for 30 minutes prior, strain, then combine all ingredients in a cocktail shaker, and pour into a martini glass. Your move, Mr. Bond.

**Ingredients**

6 juniper berries

1 cup spring water

Juice of ½ lemon

2 drops pine essential oil

1 drop peppermint essential oil

Gin and vodka, equal parts

**Intention** Skin repair, aids digestion, eases cramps, hydrates

**Lunar Phase** New

**Conjures** One serving

## ℭ The Green Faerie ℗

Transport yourself to bohemian Paris at the turn of the last century, where the birth of modern art mingled with tattered dance hall dazzle, and a heady hallucinogenic was all the rage. Crush the seeds slightly before steeping in water for 30 minutes, then strain, and pour liquid into a cocktail shaker. Add the chlorella and shake. Top your glass with vodka, and sip. This version will not have you losing your sensibilities, but rather surrendering to a state of beautified bliss, light as a little emerald pixie.

**Ingredients**

1 teaspoon anise seed

1 teaspoon fennel seed

½ teaspoon chamomile flowers

¼ teaspoon coriander seeds

1 pinch chlorella

1 cup spring water

Vodka

**Intention** Ease bloating, calm, elevate mood, feel energized

**Lunar Phase** Waning

**Conjures** One serving

## ℭ Venus Rising ℗

Rose, ruled by the goddess of love herself, has been regarded as primary medicine, a symbol of strength, and a supreme beautifier throughout the ages. Bearing gifts of love and beauty, she also grants happiness and heightens psychic awareness. Much like a woman, she is to be inhaled, anointed by, consumed, gazed upon, and adored. This voluptuous potion mingles her ample charms with the lush gifts of the pomegranate, adding a splash of your preferred bubbly to conjure a sultry Midsummer's eve any time it tickles your fancy. Make the tea first, allow it to cool, then mix it in a cocktail shaker with the rosewater and pomegranate concentrate. Pour into coupes and top with champagne.

### Ingredients

**Rose Tea**

1 tablespoon rose petals

1 teaspoon rose hips

1 cup moon water *(p. 18)*

**Cocktail**

1–2 tablespoons rose water

1 teaspoon pomegranate concentrate

A splash (or more) of champagne

**Intention** Love, lust, beauty, attraction

**Lunar Phase** Full

**Conjures** Two cocktails

## Rose Crystals, Ice Cubes

Adorn your beauty cocktails with pirate's treasure! Gorgeous sparkling gems, glistening with starlight and containing precious secrets: love crystals and a sprinkling of enchanted petals to light up your libations with festive magick.

### Ingredients

Moon water *(p. 18)*

3 pieces of rose quartz

3 pieces of pink tourmaline

Handful of rose petals

**Intention** Love, beauty, attraction

**Lunar Phase** Full

**Conjures** Twelve ice cube crystals

Place rose quartz and pink tourmaline in a large glass jar filled with moon water. Set it outside to soak up the nearly-full moonlight, and the first rays of daylight. Using an ice cube tray or mold (try the gemstone or heart-shaped ones!) sprinkle a few dried rose petals in each mold, strain the infused moon water carefully over the petals, and pop it in the freezer to set.

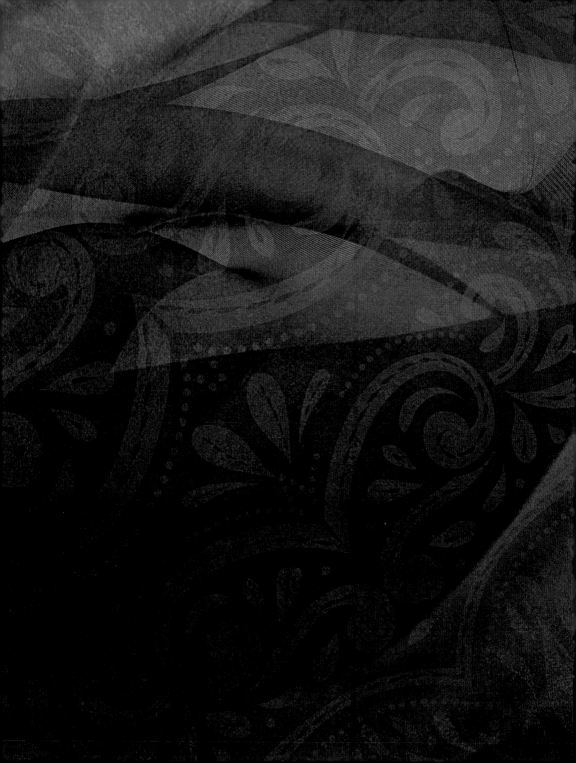

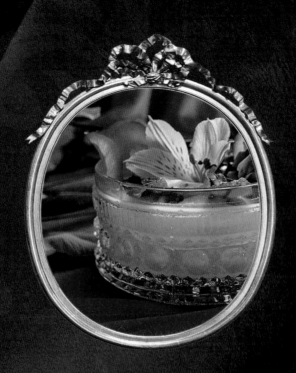

# Index of Ingredients

H ere is where the treasure is kept; hidden from curious glances, housed in myriad glamour vessels, and watched over by spirits, they grow in strength by the minute. A feast of fortune for the senses, your secret trove of magickal helpers are always ready for action. Leaves, petals, barks, nectars, and the all-powerful roots come to play with us in a joyful romp through ancient herbalist traditions from all over the globe, creating the most effective beauty potions around, to be consumed as elixirs and lovingly applied to your body.

Each ingredient found in this book is listed here, detailing its beautifying as well as magickal properties. Some you have on hand, some will be new to you. It is key to use only the highest quality potion ingredients, organic, environmentally sustainable, wildcrafted wherever possible, so please check the Resources section (p. 235) for my favorite, trusted online suppliers. Begin by gathering ingredients for the potions that beguile the most, then add to your stash whenever you can. You will find that certain potions call to you at certain times, so don't be in a flurry about making them all at once—that would be impossible! Pick one or two first, take your time, use your intuition, and enjoy the experience of concocting each new one as you desire it. Ingredients can be pricey, but once you've procured them, by all means use them: you will never have to be concerned with shelf life when you actively concoct, and then the really sexy part happens—you get to enjoy them. Savor every luscious drop!

**Abyssinian oil** With its unique molecular structure, this native Mediterranean oil boasts a high percentage of fatty acids that aid in moisturizing, cell-communicating, and protecting against heat damage, all with anti-inflammatory benefits. Even with its wild dose of moisture, it remains easily absorbed and light, making it a fabulous choice for fine hair and oily or combination skin. A relative of the mustard plant, the highly protective vibration of Mars is present, granting courage along with creation magick.

**Aloe vera** Known as the "medicine plant," lunar aloe carries the magick of protection and luck. It contains anti-inflammatory hormones which heal wounds and effectively treats conditions such a psoriasis, eczema and acne. It is a great choice of moisturizer for oily skin, and has a firming, de-puffing effect on the face and eyes. The gel and extract are used for different potions, but have equal benefits.

**Almond oil** This velvety oil is known for healing, both internally and when applied to skin. It is rich in precious vitamin E which repairs damaged skin, lessens fine lines while preventing new ones, protects against UV damage, and feeds you from head to toe. Magically, almond brings wealth and protection. They are ruled by air, which gives potions a lightness of energy surrounding the intellect, reminding you to ease up on the kind of worrying that wreaks havoc on your face.

**Amber** Sacred to Freya, gorgeous amber is a gift of the sun, radiating joy and life-force energy. It has a cleansing effect on the blood, boosting circulation, which carries oxygen and nutrients to the skin. It also strengthens tissue.

**Apple cider vinegar** In its raw form, apple cider vinegar is a natural tonic with the ability to lower blood sugar, lessen sweet cravings, aids in weight loss, improves digestion, and increases the bodies' ability to absorb nutrients. Topically, it removes dead skin cells, balances pH levels, and imparts shine to both skin and hair. Naturally, it contains all the magick of its mother fruit, the apple.

**Apple** Said to give perpetual youth to the gods, apples were revered throughout the ancient world as offerings to beauty, love, and lust. Ruled by Venus, and sacred to Freya, they also are potent bringers of peace and good health. Apple is rich in natural alpha hydroxy acids that exfoliate both mature and acne-prone skin brilliantly, shedding dull dead skin and revealing a fresh new layer. It is also high in nutrients and antioxidants, which are not only crucial to youthful skin, but are required even more post-exfoliation, when new skin is vulnerable and needs nourishment and protection. For this reason, pairing apple with a rich base oil is an excellent choice.

**Aquamarine** Bathed in the healing powers of the ancient seas, the "mermaid stone" promotes well-being, cleansing, and tranquility. Its mineral content makes it a classic beauty stone known for its powers of rejuvenation.

**Arrowroot** A nutritive alternative to cornstarch, arrowroot was named for its ability to treat arrow wounds long ago, thus carrying healing magick. It absorbs excess oil, is gluten-free, and contains vitamins, minerals, and phytonutrients that keep the scalp and skin well fed, and leave hair shiny and manageable.

**Ashwagandha** This ancient Ayurvedic adaptogen herb has been long revered for its abilities to lessen stress, boost immunity, support brain function, increase energy, build physical stamina, and help with restful sleep. It holds the magick of the horse, representing great strength and sexuality.

**Avocado** Rich and sensual, avocado oil has long been associated with beauty and love magick. Ripe with good fats, this Venusian gem is an excellent moisturizer high in vitamin E, fighting the signs of aging and feeding your skin while soothing inflammation and breakouts. When consumed, the creamy density of the fruit keeps you full without heaviness, and works wonders from the inside out. It is also a noted aphrodisiac.

**Baking soda** This ubiquitous kitchen refresher is a purely alkaline "salt" which not only whitens teeth, but soothes an occasional upset tummy and cleans surfaces naturally.

**Banana** The humble banana is actually an ancient sacred food in the East, closely tied to spirituality. It is said to bring luck and heighten feelings of love. Bananas also make a wonderfully rich hair treatment for their combination of a high water content and natural moisturizing oils, which help repair damaged strands and increase elasticity.

**Basil** A freshly-scented garden favorite, basil is a strong anti-inflammatory, antibacterial herb loaded with antioxidants. Topically, it soothes skin, treats acne, and gently cleanses with the magick of love, protection, and abundance. In certain circles, is even used to halt the sexual wanderings of married men!

**Bay laurel** Nibbled by ancient Greek priestesses to read prophecy, bay has long been a magickal herb of clairvoyance and wisdom. Also used for protection, healing, and strength, it is antiseptic and astringent when used in topical potions. Also a great muscle soother, it has a spicy, uplifting scent that promotes feelings of well-being, enhanced creativity, and confidence.

**Beetroot** This gorgeously hued root is loaded with vitamins A and C—so essential to health and beauty—warding off lines and wrinkles, promoting healthy cell turnover, maintaining elasticity, and keeping skin firm. Detoxifying, blood circulating, and immune-boosting, they bring pure love magick in, and are essential in supporting the root chakra.

**Besan (garbanzo flour)** This ancient Ayurvedic skin beautifier is one of my all-time faves for its gentle yet effective exfoliation powers, and the stellar nutrition it delivers to your skin. I love to use it thrice weekly, even just on its own, to lift away old cells and leave skin glowy, hydrated, and firm.

**Blackberry** Ruled by Venus, this sexy berry carries not only her beauty magick, but that of abundance and creation. They can even boost your love life! Voluptuous with antioxidants, bioflavonoids, and vitamins—most notably vitamin C—blackberries refine and feed the skin, while revving the all-important cell renewal process. Their deep hue ensures vibrant Jing energy, so vital to our inner *and* outer radiance.

**Bloodstone** Mysterious bloodstone has been valued since ancient times as a healing stone, and one that banishes negativity. It has even been known to guide one who is lost. Known to stop excessive bleeding, it has been used during childbirth and been worn by warriors for not only wounds, but to provide courage. As a beauty stone, it revs circulation, heals tissue, and possesses reparative properties, to lessen fine lines and wrinkles while it brings new blood flow to the skin.

**Blue tansy** Blue tansy is part of the chamomile family, and commonly known as Moroccan chamomile. It boasts a sweet scent and a natural hue that sirens find most attractive, along with a higher concentration of compounds than other varieties of chamomile. Like them, it soothes and calms skin while bringing forth the magick of peace and prosperity. It also moisturizes well without an oiliness, so it works well for eruptive skin, and contains antioxidants which combat premature aging. Can you substitute the more common chamomile oils? Yes, of course. They just won't be quite as potent.

**Blueberry** This luscious superfood is loaded with antioxidants, which fight both disease and visible signs of aging. Ruled by the Moon and water, blueberry offers protective energy to both our magical workings *and* our bodies.

**Borage** The Jupiter-ruled magick of borage conjures courage, heightened psychic abilities, and intense moisture. It's no wonder that Witches know borage as both Star Flower and Herb of Gladness—it can heal and protect even the most arid, cracked skin to restore a plumped and soft texture. With high amounts of gamma-linoleic acid, borage seed oil soothes eruptive skin conditions like eczema with anti-inflammatory aplomb, while strengthening the outermost layer and locking in moisture. Fair warning:

borage does not smell heavenly. Concoct together with strongly scented oils to avoid horror-filled glances in your direction.

**Brahmi** This amazing Ayurvedic oil encourages hair growth quickly and effectively. Traditionally massaged onto the scalp, it carries the magick of bestowing intellect as it eases stress, promotes restful sleep, and sharpens concentration and memory.

**Brown rice flour** This humble pantry staple becomes a beauty booster that you'll want to keep in mind: as an exfoliant it has a polishing effect that sloughs a bit deeper than the softer flours, but still remains gentle and nutritive for sensitive skin. It also can help to lighten hyperpigmentation over time. Brown rice carries the energy of both the sun and air, and magickally aids abundance, creativity, and sex, all with a protective cloak.

**Burdock root** Venus-ruled burdock is an old witch's favorite for protection, healing, and warding off negativity. When consumed, burdock boosts immunity and removes toxins from the blood, which supports kidneys and the lymphatic system. Naturally detoxifying, this powerful root also eases skin condition such as acne and eczema, while fighting wrinkles and promoting healthy hair.

**Cacao** Ruled by fire, cacao is a magickal food of love and riches. It is incredibly high in antioxidants (which prevent cell and tissue damage), with iron, magnesium, protein, minerals, essential fatty acids, and calcium— all of which contribute to supple skin, shiny hair, and strong nails, making it a superior beauty food blessed with the enchantments of a mood-elevating aphrodisiac. This love food increases blood flow and serotonin levels, enhancing mood and stirring sexual desire.

**Cactus water** Cactus water comes from the fruit of the prickly pear cactus, and is loaded with antioxidants, vitamins A, C, E, iron, calcium, and has anti-inflammatory properties. Immensely hydrating, it has a fruity, light flavor, and not a trace of sugar to be found. In fact, it actually *lowers* blood sugar, making it a sublime beauty sip. Magickally, it is highly protective.

**Candelilla wax** Candelilla wax is a plant-based alternative to beeswax which creates a buttery, easily blended balm. The gift of a native Mexican shrub, it is highly emollient, easily absorbed, and rich in nutrients. It also has a lovely, sweet scent when heated.

**Calendula** Also known as marigold, calendula flowers are ruled by fire, yet offer soothing, curative comforts to the skin, and can be extremely helpful for rashes, inflammation, dry patches, and other irritations. Honored by the ancient Egyptians for their rejuvenating powers, they have been known to bring forth protection, prophetic dreams, and heightened psychic insight.

**Carrot seed & carrot root** Fiery carrots are lusty bringers of sexual desire. Mars-ruled, they contain active anti-aging warriors, but there is a distinction between the seed oil and the root extract. The seed oil provides a natural sunscreen, is loaded with antioxidants, and amps up circulation which gives the skin a healthy glow. The root is full of vitamin A, and does wonders as a natural Retinol. Together they make quite a pair!

**Cashew** Ruled by the Sun's fire, creamy cashews bring forth money magick. High in beauty fats, cashews are also rich in nutrients, protein, minerals, and vitamin E—a highly effective oil which repairs skin, including wrinkles. They are a good natural source of selenium, an antioxidant which helps to protect cells from damage, thereby preventing accelerated ageing in skin.

**Castile soap** Conjured from plant-derived oils, castile soap is a gentle way to cleanse skin, hair, and surfaces without chemicals. Safe and effective for even the most sensitive skin, it makes an excellent base for beauty potions, deriving magick and benefits from the blend of oils used.

**Castor** The rich, syrupy oil of the castor plant is an important ingredient in skincare, though it is often overlooked. Due to its extra-thick texture, it takes a while to absorb into skin, but is entirely worth the wait. The acids contained in the oil actually inhibit bacteria while allowing moisture to penetrate into the skin, making it favorable to sensitive, acne-prone, and aging skin. It has a potent softening and smoothing effect, while granting protection and dispelling negative energy.

**Catnip** What could be nicer than an herb that makes cats happy? Ruled by Venus and sacred to Bast, this one, naturally, brings love, beauty, and joy to felines and humans alike with its magic *and* its delightful scent. Used for calming nerves, catnip also has a mild sedative effect, and is helpful for the monthly woes of cramping and mood swings. It also works wonders for easing digestion and fever. Used topically, catnip heals an irritated scalp while acting as an anti-inflammatory for skin.

**Cats claw** Any plant named for a feline talon has *got* to be magickal—and this beautiful flowering South American native vine is just that. Prized for its anti-inflammatory and immune-strengthening powers, it also is held in high shamanic regard as a life-giving herb that connects the body to the spirt, and gives balance to both. It is said to heighten psychic abilities, bring forth abundance, and enhance vision quests.

**Cayenne** Sublimely spicy cayenne is commonly used to promote beauty from the inside out for its anti-inflammatory properties, its ability to support both detoxification and the immune system, and its thermogenic (metabolism boosting) powers. Externally, however, cayenne increases blood flow and circulation to the skin, making it too irritating in many instances, but effective in giving a plumped effect to the lips.

**Cedarwood** Solar-powered cedarwood stimulates hair follicles by increasing circulation to the scalp, and has a natural thickening ability. A tree of purification, it also holds healing and money magick. I find it also has a grounding effect, locked inside the wisdom of the forest.

**Celtic sea salt** This is a potent detoxifier that is rich in all precious trace minerals. It is harvested by ancient methods, and left in its natural state, bringing pure sea magic straight into your bath. Interestingly, salt is ruled by earth, which also gives it a grounding, protective magick.

**Chamomile** A darling little flower with magick to spare, chamomile soothes and provides tranquility during an emotional storm, and helps to clear negativity. But don't be fooled by its sweet scent and subtle allure: chamomile softens and moisturizes your skin beautifully while *seriously* attracting love and abundance.

**Champagne** Could there be a more unabashed bombshell delight? Ah, but lunar champagne *also* has a few beauty secrets floating inside those starlit bubbles: it contains the significant antioxidant power of the grape, tartaric acid to even skin tone, and has both antibacterial and anti-inflammatory benefits.

**Charcoal, activated** This powdered powerhouse cleans and detoxifies skin deeply, making it an excellent choice for acne-prone and oily skin, and helpful for any skin type that can use a deep cleanse. Its texture will give a more vigorous manual exfoliation than most flours, so those with sensitive skin may want to avoid the sloughing and stick with its bacteria-lifting masque benefits. Make sure to buy vegetarian/vegan, as activated charcoal can sometimes contain bone ash.

**Chia seed/black chia** Easily digested, chia is a complete protein designed to hydrate. It is rich in omega fatty acids, fiber, and minerals, making it an excellent staple to your beauty food diet. As an oil, it is rich in omega-3 oils, making it a powerhouse moisturizer for even very dry and irritated skin. It has the ability to heal damaged skin (including wrinkles) while helping to maintain a strong moisture barrier on the epidermis.

**Chlorella** This jade-hued beauty is an amazing source of clean plant protein and vital nutrients that boost the immune system, lower blood sugar and cholesterol, and fight degenerative disease. It holds the magick of water, and is used topically to promote collagen production, increase elasticity, and reduce redness. Best part? You can't beat her for firming skin!

**Cinnamon** Amorous cinnamon ignites the fires of both love and money, while cleansing and increasing circulation to both your skin and scalp. The increased blood flow brings life to the skin, for a glowing radiance; for hair, it stimulates new growth. Cinnamon also has anti-inflammatory, antioxidant, and warming properties to strengthen and beautify from the inside out. It also regulates blood sugar. If possible, buy pure Ceylon cinnamon—it is a healthier option, particularly if you consume it regularly.

**Cloudberry** This great Nordic beauty berry is rich in Omega fats that make skin fresh and dewy, with healing properties to keep moisture intact and wrinkles at bay. Norse berries have the strength to withstand fierce winters as well as intense solar power, making them ideal beauty ingredients, particularly for dry and maturing skin.

**Coconut** Sweet, buttery coconut oil is known for its beautifying fats, but is also a bacteria-fighting warrior that prevents viruses and other harmful pathogens from attacking. Though it can be somewhat clogging to the skin, and is therefore best kept off the face, it makes a stellar hair treatment. Coconut oil tames frizz, prevents protein loss, adds shine, controls dandruff, and deeply penetrates hair for superior conditioning. It makes a great tooth cleanser, too, due to its antimicrobial and antifungal prowess, removes eye makeup gently, and packs a wallop as a natural (and *very* pleasurable) lubricant. Add a dollop to your Kitchen Witchery, and you've got it made: coconut oil adds a bit of beauty fat necessary to help absorb dark greens. This lunar ruled gem also heightens spirituality and psychic awareness.

**Coconut nectar** Blessed with the magick of the coconut, the sweet sap of this lunar gift raises psychic awareness and promotes spirituality while treating you to a mineral rich, low-glycemic sweetness. It works particularly well paired with fruit flavors.

**Coffee/coffee bean extract** Fire-ruled coffee is a favorite brew for many, but it can wreak havoc on your beauty. Though it can certainly stimulate the conscious mind and give us a little boost in small doses, as a diuretic it is extremely dehydrating to the skin, causing fine lines and wrinkles to become more visible, and, eventually, deeper. It also causes bloating. Adding to the mix, caffeine triggers stress hormones, which can cause breakouts and other eruptions. However, when used topically, caffeine becomes a unique combination of antioxidant, diuretic (skin-smoother), and vasoconstrictor (puffiness and dark spot reducer), which can improve skin's appearance immensely. Best to slather on than to swig.

**Comfrey** Comfrey heals skin, promotes new hair growth, and fortifies with rich nutritive fats, vitamins, and minerals. Magickally, it protects and brings forth abundance.

**Coriander** As an ancient Ayurvedic healing herb, these bitter seeds of the cilantro plant have long been used to grant good health, but also to increase love and lust. Ruled by Mars and fire, coriander is most commonly used to aid digestion, reduce anxiety, ease bloat, and help you to sleep.

**Cardamom** Sensual and warm, zesty cardamom boosts circulation, contains potent antioxidants, helps with weight loss and maintenance, quells anxiety, fights disease, treats skin allergies and improves complexion. It is a gift of Venus, infused with the magick of love, lust, beauty, and protection.

**Clary sage** is a wonderful antidepressant and slightly sedative oil that produces feelings of euphoria. It is also antibacterial and highly protective from a magick standpoint. *Do not use clary sage if you are pregnant.*

**Clear quartz** One of the most common Witches crystals, clear quartz has many magickal uses: it amplifies intention, helps to attune you to your higher self, aids in attaining spiritual growth, helps to expand the mind, protects, and heals. Symbolic of both the Moon and water, it is highly effective during ritual—just keep your intentions clear and positive, and it will intensify any energy present.

**Cranberry** Ruled by water and bearing protection energy, cranberries are loaded with hydration, high levels of antioxidants, and a perfect Omega fats ratio that allows for amazing absorption into the skin. These tart little treats provide lots of vitamin C and fiber, are excellent at detoxifying, and can keep infection at bay.

**Cucumber extract/cucumber seed oil** Cucumber is ruled by the Moon and water, bringing peace and healing alongside significant beauty benefits. Gentle and soothing, the extract relieves irritated skin and has a mildly astringent effect, making it an excellent ingredient for oily and eruption-prone complexions. Rich in antioxidants and silica, it relieves puffiness while firming and helping to diminish fine lines and wrinkles. Cucumber seed oil is rich in vitamin E and phytosterols, which encourage cell regeneration, new growth, elasticity and a strong moisture barrier. It also repairs brittle and peeling nails, and makes an excellent light moisturizer.

**Cumin/black cumin seed oil** Fiery cumin is a highly protective seed that can aid in anti-theft and exorcism magick. It is also said to help ensure fidelity and inspire lust when consumed. High in antioxidants, it also helps digestion, eases bloat, treats headaches, and stabilizes blood sugar. Topically, cumin strengthens hair, contains the skin repair sorcery of vitamin E, and nourishes with beautifying essential minerals. Regulates sebum production.

**Cypress** Sacred to Aphrodite, the highly protective cypress is a symbol of immortality. Possessing the energies of healing, comfort, protection, and longevity, cypress revs circulation to detoxify and get the blood flowing. As such, it makes an excellent treatment for acne, cellulite, and varicose veins. Earthy cypress also eases anxiety and promotes restful sleep.

**Damiana** Ruled by fire, lusty damiana has long been revered by witches as an aphrodisiac. It elevates your stamina, enhances mood, and is an excellent tonic for overworked kidneys. A lesser known gift of this sexy plant is its ability to induce visions.

**Dates** Long presented as offerings to both the gods and the departed, dates are tokens of strength and spirituality. They make excellent low glycemic natural sweeteners rich in vitamins and minerals, and support fresh skin with antioxidants.

**Elder flower** Elder flower is known for fighting colds and flu effectively, but it also provides a bit of beauty sorcery: these delicate faerie blossoms tighten skin, refine pores, soothes the scalp, and effectively moisturizes dry hair, all with the magic of healing and protection.

**Emerald** Long considered a powerful anti-aging stone, emerald has powerful rejuvenating energies to help increase elasticity, reduce fine lines, and prevent eruptions.

**Eucalyptus** The uplifting scent of the eucalyptus clears the mind and energetically detoxifies the air, but this native Australian lunar plant also has great healing powers: it can ward off a cold or flu (and relieve symptoms once you have them,) reduce pain, lower inflammation, and cleanse with its antimicrobial and antibacterial capacities. Naturally it carries the magick of healing and protection.

**Fennel** Fire-powered fennel actually bears the gift of soothing, cloaked in protection. Anise-flavored fennel eases tummy troubles, aids digestion, reduces inflammation (and the dreaded bloat!) and revs metabolism while providing key vitamins and minerals.

**Fir** The earthy scent of the forest lives in fir, bringing tree wisdom and magick to everything it touches, along with cleansing, protection, and healing. It's antibacterial, anti-inflammatory, soothing powers also make it an excellent topical potion ingredient.

**Frankincense** Quite possibly the most effective of all ancient beauty secrets, the Solar fire of frankincense glows like no other. A powerful protective offering, it also holds high spiritual vibrations and the power to banish. Indeed, it is an age-fighting superstar which keeps wrinkles away, tightens pores, and visibly lifts and firms the skin. Its scent is absolutely swoon-worthy.

**French green clay** Earthy green clay is a gentle but powerful detoxifying clay suitable for all skin types, that firms and tones, stimulates circulation, cleanses, and exfoliates. It is mined in France, untreated, keeping both its naturally beautiful hue, as well as its potency, intact.

**Garam masala** This delightful spice blend hails from Southeast Asia, bringing a heavenly scent and a bit of heat to everything it touches. Usually, it is a combination of black pepper, cinnamon, fennel, cardamom, nutmeg, bay, cumin, coriander, and a bit of chili pepper, bringing forth the healing powers and magick of each spice.

**Geranium** Classic garden geranium is indeed a highly protective friend of the Witch (not to mention a beloved nibble of our beautiful deer friends!) that also carries the magick of creativity, good health, and love. It relieves anxiety, eases depression, and has considerable antibacterial, anti-inflammatory, and antioxidant benefits.

**Gin** Fire-powered and ruled by the Sun, this spirit contains the magick of the berry it comes from: juniper. It has been used in protection and exorcism spells, to increase male sexual potency, and, interestingly, to promote good health. Indeed, it is a good choice for imbibing. Gin is (relatively) low-calorie and low-sugar, contains beautifying vitamin C and antioxidants, reduces inflammation and helps digestion.

**Ginger** A great power root, ginger is known for its fire magick, protection, and ability to bring good health. A warming spice, it increases circulation, relieves nausea and lessens pain.

**Ginseng** This ancient Chinese medicinal herb is fantastic for tightening, toning, and brightening the skin. A protective, fiery Solar root, it has magickal properties of beauty, love, lust, and granting wishes: no wonder it boosts collagen formation!

**Glycerin** Sweet vegetable glycerin is a light, clear syrup that acts as a humectant—useful for both a beauty potion and a sore throat. Like all humectants, however, it requires blending with an occlusive (protective barrier) such as avocado or olive oil to work properly, by preventing moisture loss.

**Goji** Delicious, potent goji has long been revered in Traditional Chinese Medicine (TCM) as a healing fruit. It balances the body, strengthens the kidneys, assists joints and bones, and improves eye health—all with massive amounts of vitamin C and an ancient reputation for its age-delaying magick.

**Grape** Grapes are water fruits that hold the magic of both fertility and prosperity, making them fabulous consorts when it comes to creative endeavors. What's more, they have beauty benefits to spare: rich in antioxidants and flavonoids, they promote new cellular growth, reduce fine lines, increase elasticity, restore collagen, impart sheen, and provide UV protection. Red grapes are ruled by the Sun, white by the Moon.

**Grapefruit** Ruled by the Sun, this bright, juicy sphere brings the magick of strength and purification, along with an unexpected dash of intuitive water sorcery. It contains high levels of vitamin C and antioxidants, eases digestion and stabilizes blood sugar, and provides significant hydration. Your skin is also in good hands, with the added perk of repairing and preventing UV damage from the inside.

**Grapeseed** Mineral-rich grape-seed oil feeds the scalp with proteins and vitamin E but is light enough to impart shine on all types of hair, and moisture to all types of skin, without heaviness or greasiness. The fertile seeds of lunar Bacchanalian grapes contain flavonoids which strengthen collagen and bones, along with heightened mental abilities and money magick.

**Green tea extract** Known as "liquid jade," green tea is protective and healing, with the energy of love whether new or renewed. It contains high levels of antioxidants which can slow down the signs of aging. Its gentle astringent properties can help shrink blood vessels below the surface, which can lessen swelling and dark circles under the eyes with long-term effects.

**Helichrysum** Known as the Everlasting Flower, helichrysum has long been heralded for its ability to fight fine lines and wrinkles. Though highly active, it calms and soothes skin—particularly after being in the sun—and is an effective spot treatment for blemishes and eruptions, all the while seducing you with its lovely floral scent. It has great efficacy in improving the appearance of fine lines and wrinkles, while keeping new ones at bay for as long as possible by promoting cell regeneration.

**Hibiscus** Revered by the ancient Egyptians for its hydrating prowess, hibiscus is also immensely effective for keeping skin firm and increasing elasticity. It contains inhibitors that protect skin from the breaking down of elastin—a key factor in keeping skin lifted. It is also rich in vitamin C, an essential nutrient in boosting collagen, which is beneficial to both skin and hair.

**Himalayan pink salt** Mined 5,000 feet deep below its namesake mountain range, Himalayan pink salt was subject to enormous pressure over millions of years and is over 99% pure. The greater the amount of pressure, the more superior the state of order within the crystalline structure of the salt—also making the higher quality versions pricier, but worth it, as they are pure and assimilate easily into the body. As a smooth yet highly effective exfoliant, it is also a potent soak containing major minerals that will absorb into skin as it detoxifies and soothes aches.

**Horny goat weed (Barrenwort)** Touted for its male sexual health benefits, this herb is also sometimes used for joint pain and to ease the discomfort of osteoporosis. Here, we call upon the Witches herb to heighten sexual desire, and improve erectile function.

**Horsetail** Horsetail is an ancient remedy for healing, which is also used in beauty potions for soothing, repairing, and firming skin with its high concentration of silica. It is used in serpent magick and to promote fertility and creativity.

**Hyaluronic acid /HA** Despite having "acid" in its name, this beautifying dew is not an intense exfoliator, but rather a naturally-occurring polysaccharide found in the human body that diminishes as we age. It is responsible for cushioning our joints, nerves, skin, hair, and eyes, acting as a lubricant. This is what gives our younger skin a plumped, soft look. By adding it to our potions, it visually fills in fine lines and gives skin a youthful appearance. As a humectant, it works best with an occlusive oil (like avocado, olive, or cacao butter, for instance) to create a protective moisture barrier.

**Hyssop** A relative of the mint plant, hyssop is used primarily as an herb of purification. Ruled by fire and expansive Jupiter, it is also highly protective, particularly in banishing and shielding against intense forms of negativity.

**Jasmine** Known as "The Queen of The Night," sensual jasmine is an intoxicating aphrodisiac that knows a thing about beauty. A brilliant oil for reducing fine lines and strengthening skin's elasticity, jasmine also helps fade scars and hyper-pigmentation. It strengthens the scalp and roots for healthy new growth, while imparting a gloriously protective shine to the length of your tresses.

**Juniper** Gorgeous, fiery juniper berries are tiny powerhouses ruled by the Sun, and full of his vitality. They are filled with protective, virile, energy that promotes good health, and are used in exorcism spells. Juniper will heighten psychic abilities and clears away negativity.

**Kale** This detoxifying, immune-boosting superstar offers splendid amounts of iron, calcium, vitamin A, and beautifying minerals that support every inch of your foxy self, with the added coup of conjuring money magick.

**Kelp** Another sacred gift of the oceans, a variety of reddish-brown seaweed that grows in lush forests beneath the sea, revered as a protective energy, and believed to bring happiness. Ruled by the Moon, kelp is highly nutritious, but also possesses detoxifying properties. It contains potassium, iron, and niacin, which keeps you glowing by increasing blood circulation, brightening the skin, and providing hydration. An ample dose of vitamin C stimulates collagen from the inside out, for potent age-delaying results.

**Kombucha** Who would imagine something fermented could be so sexy? But it is. Fizzy, fun kombucha is the love child of tea, fermentation, and a retinue of add-ins that increase its potency. Probiotic, immune-boosting, and rich in antioxidants, kombucha makes a fabulous statement when added to a beauty cocktail.

**Lavender** Lunar-ruled lavender soothes, calms anxiety, and brings peace. It also protects hair from thinning and loss while simultaneously aiding in new growth, and makes a fantastic skin treatment thanks to its antibacterial powers. Known as "Elf Leaf," it holds powers of love, peacefulness, protection, and longevity—not surprising given its namesake!

**Lapis lazuli** Lapis, also known as "the truth stone," conveyed the wisdom of Isis in ancient Egypt, accompanied Sumerian goddess Inanna into the underworld, and was used to convey messages of love and good luck in the royal courts of 18th century France and England. It opens up your ability to communicate effectively, and activates the throat chakra.

**Lapsang souchong** Tea leaves and buds smoked over a pine fire to create a very sultry tea, prized for its smooth, dark flavor. Tea is ruled by fire, bringing courage and abundance. This one adds a touch of sublimely sexy allure to potions.

**Lemon** Bright, zesty lemon is a lunar-ruled fruit of love, happiness, and cleansing. Its vitamin C kick helps to boost immunity, while its high level of calcium strengthens teeth and bones. A natural detoxifier, lemon cheers and energizes while clarifying skin and lightening hyperpigmentation.

**Lepidolite** Lilac-hued lepidolite naturally and effectively lowers anxiety, decreases feelings of stress, and has the power to bestow serenity and bring the bearer into the present moment.

**Licorice root** Prized by the ancient Egyptians, licorice root is a beauty booster that is easily overlooked, but shouldn't be. It is ruled by Venus, after all! Licorice root does wonders to repair, firm and promote radiance in the skin, and promotes hair growth, all while bringing forth love, lust, and beauty magick.

**Lime** Solar-powered lime carries love, protection, and healing magick. Rich in vitamin C and antioxidants, limes support beauty from the inside, as well as being a potent topical treatment. They brighten and tone the skin, fight the visible signs of aging, and act as an astringent.

**Lion's mane** Named for its resemblance to that fabulous feline crowning glory, this medicinal mushroom is an ancient superfood prized for its antioxidant, anti-inflammatory, and immune boosting powers. It also sharpens focus, improves cognitive function, and reduces anxiety.

**Longan fruit powder** Longan is used in Traditional Chinese Medicine (TCM) as a spleen, heart, and blood tonic, which translates into youth and vitality. High in vitamin C, longan is also touted for bringing vitality to the skin, both internally and topically.

**Lotus flower/lotus root** A sacred ancient offering to the gods, lotus is looked upon as a symbol of life. It brings protection, healing, fertility, rebirth, and it is even said to hold the power of breaking locks. Ruled by the Moon and water, the lotus is known as a type of water lily, providing moisture to dry, parched skin. It also helps to balance the skin's oil content, making it an excellent choice for all skin types. Its vibration also adds a bit of kick to your sex life.

**Maca** The wild South American maca is revered as a superfood for its nutrients and adaptogenic quality, as well as its lust and fertility magick. Maca is used for boosting libido in both men and women, but it has a particular strength as a male sexual tonic: boosting healthy sperm, increasing energy, balancing hormones, and heightening sex drive.

**Maple syrup** This Jupiter-ruled nectar of the sacred maple tree carries their love and money magick alongside the ability to increase longevity. Indeed, though a natural sugar and therefore not suited to everyone, maple syrup is rich in vitamins, minerals, and antioxidants—making this a lower-glycemic, healthier beauty choice.

**Matcha** Matcha, a super-charged form of green tea, is the star of graceful Japanese ceremonial rites that are performed to honor mindfulness and presence. It is an antioxidant powerhouse with tremendous health benefits, which, when applied topically, is also a beauty bombshell that assists cell rejuvenation, provides UV protection, and acts as an anti-inflammatory. Magically, it is ruled by fire, giving courage, assisting in money matters, and elevating the conscious mind.

**Magnesium** An oft-overlooked, but necessary mineral, magnesium is not only important in the diet (good sources are dark chocolate, avocados, legumes, nuts, seeds) but is a fabulous addition to a bath. Absorbed through the skin, magnesium soothes aches, sore muscles and joints, instills a sense of calm, beautifies skin, and helps to lull you to sleep.

**Mango** Sensual, fiery mango gifts us with love and sex magick surrounded by protection energy. Loaded with beauty nutrients like vitamins A, B6, C, beta carotene and folates (and dense in calories—be careful!) mango is a lush and sexy addition to potions.

**Meadowfoam** From the flowering beauty of damp woodlands and tide pools comes meadowfoam seed oil, an age-fighting warrior made of 98% fatty acid. Similar to the skin's natural sebum, it creates a protective outer layer which locks moisture in while simultaneously delivering it deep into your epidermis. High in antioxidants, it also has superior firming abilities, feels like velvet, and carries the magick of both water and earth.

**Medicinal mushroom blend** Lunar-ruled and marvelously earthy, mushrooms are one of the most potent superfoods we have been given. A good medicinal blend will contain chaga, lion's mane, turkey tail, and reishi—with potentially a few other gems in there—for detoxifying, strengthening your immune system, improving brain function, revitalizing the body, and building strength and endurance.

**Mica powder** Mineral mica powder is a blend of minerals that make sparkles. Though completely natural, it has come under fire for labor policies and sustainability issues. Synthetic mica powder is made in a lab but from natural materials and does not contain plastic. There are companies now citing that their natural mica is ethically sourced—please see Resources (p. 235)—but I would still recommend using it sparingly as to not deplete natural resources.

**Moonstone** This shimmering, otherworldly stone awakens feminine energies such as intuition, creativity, nurturing, protection, and healing. It also absorbs the energy of the moon herself as she waxes and wanes.

**Moroccan red clay** This rich red clay draws impurities from your skin, while adding a stabilizing earth energy. It deeply cleans pores, firms and tightens, promotes cellular regeneration, increases elasticity, and brightens skin.

**Mugwort** Ruled by Venus and sacred to Diana, this Witch's favorite is a must-have. Traditionally burned for protection, I also find it incredibly strengthening. Internally, it eases tummy woes, loosens joints, and boosts energy. *Do not ingest mugwort if you are pregnant.*

**Mustard seed** Mustard seed is widely used in Ayurvedic practice to ignite the digestive "fire," reduce pain and inflammation, and slow the growth of certain diseases. Added to a bath or skin blend, it has age-delay effects, heals irritations, and is delightfully warming. It carries the magick of fire, creativity, protection, and increased mental prowess.

**Myrrh** The female consort of frankincense is surely lovely, lunar myrrh. It has a similar high spiritual vibration to its solar partner, also bringing potent healing and protective energy. As they share anti-aging properties, they make an unbeatable beauty pair. Not surprisingly, they were both revered in ancient Egypt for their magick.

**Myrtle** Blessed with an uplifting scent, myrtle revives the spirit, while it's cleansing properties keep pores clear and skin refreshed. This lovely herb carries love, money, and creative magick, as it promotes youthful beauty.

**Nectarine** Venusian nectarine is named for the Greek word meaning "drink of the gods"—one taste and you will agree—the sweet, juicy flesh is pure pleasure. Fiber-rich and filled with nutrients, these delightful fruits cleanse as they hydrate, feeding your mood and your glow.

**Neroli** With its sweet and cheerful orange blossom scent, Neroli is both sublimely sensual *and* a beauty bombshell. It has the ability to balance the skin; hydrating and fighting the signs of aging while simultaneously calming and clearing irritated skin. As such, it works equally well on mature or oily skin. A fire-powered gift of the sun, Neroli brings gifts of love, luck, and money along with heightened abilities for divination.

**Nettle** Mars-ruled nettle is a wild little powerhouse used for banishing negativity and protection—but it also conjures lust and healing. What's more, nettle is an intense beauty food adding gloss and new growth to the hair, firmness and clarity to the skin, and eliminating bloat.

**Nordic spruce** With an average life span of 10,000 years, the majestic Norway spruce is closely associated with longevity and strength. It has been trusted for its healing properties for centuries, and is known for its ability to heal dry, cracked skin with age-defying powers of rejuvenation. It also provides gentle cleansing and astringent benefits, and an enchanted faerie forest scent.

**Nordic berry powder** A wildcrafted blend of Nordic blueberry, bilberry, black currant, and blackberry, this mystic powder adds a potent energy/ mood/ immune boost to your elixirs, with high levels of antioxidants, phytonutrients, minerals and vitamins. Infused into your skincare, they protect against wrinkles, dullness, and loss of elasticity while revitalizing with the magick of protection, love, beauty, and sexuality.

**Nutmeg** Fiery, Jupiter-ruled nutmeg prevents hair loss and encourages new growth while keeping tresses shiny. Anti-bacterial and anti-microbial, it works wonders on oily skin, imparts a healthy glow, and even fights wrinkles. It is also highly valued for its ability to open up our psychic awareness.

**Oats** Earthy oats are gifts of Venus that not only contain her beauty magick, but also a generous dollop of abundance. Used topically, they calm and soothe irritated skin and act as a humectant packed with beauty minerals copper, biotin, magnesium, and vitamin B.

**Olive oil** This ancient Mediterranean beauty treatment is often overlooked due to its thick, viscous, texture. Though this makes it slower to absorb into the skin, that's the point really. As a nutrient-dense occlusive oil, it creates a protective barrier to keep moisture in the skin. It also contains squalene which is an amazing hydrator. Olive brings love, protection, healing, creativity, and lust.

**Onyx** Closely associated with the root chakra, onyx is considered a stone of power. Its vibration purifies the skin, helping to heal inflammation, infections, and sunburn.

**Orange carnelian** Revered by the ancient Egyptians for its feminine power, orange carnelian is ruled by fire, and ignites the inner flame of passion by opening the sacral chakra.

**Oregano** The oil of peaceful oregano is actually a highly potent antibiotic and anti-fungal treatment both internally and when used topically. It kills bacteria, eases gastrointestinal woes, and soothes the respiratory system.

**Passionflower** Though its name suggests more active bedroom rituals, Venus-ruled passionflower promotes peaceful slumber. Calming and harmonious, it can also quell anxiety and soothe skin.

**Patchouli** Feminine and earthy, patchouli is more than a ubiquitous festival oil: it holds strong lust magick! It also brings forth creativity and abundance, while providing relaxation, easing depressive feelings, and treating dry/irritated skin conditions.

**Pau d'arco** This Amazonian native is revered for its ability to heighten spirituality related to healing and bringing forth power. Physically, its bark strengthens the immune system, kills bacteria, and fights infection, making it an important addition to healing potions.

**Peach** Nectarine's sister fruit is a native of China and considered sacred. Lushly emollient and rich in vitamin C, peach is a powerful and pleasurable age-delay beautifier which bears the magickal gifts of love, happiness, wisdom, and good health.

**Peony root** Insert text

**Peppermint/mint** Delightfully cooling peppermint is actually ruled by fire, and as such excels in bringing forth action as well as being a passionate love and lust herb. It adds a dash of cooling, healing, and purifying energy, with a stimulating power that freshens skin *and* lifts your mood.

**Pine/pine bark extract** The great Mars-ruled pine is revered for its healing and fertility magick, as well as being a powerful protector. This translates to your skin: it shields your skin from damaging rays while strengthening the skin barrier, acts as an inflammatory, and is high in antioxidants.

**Pine pollen** Another gift of the sacred pine tree, pine pollen is effective in increasing energy, boosting immunity, and has age-delay prowess to spare. Gentlemen, take note: this magick dust is also used in Chinese medicine to increase male sexual and athletic performance.

**Pineapple** Solar-powered pineapple is filled with fire magick, as well as the powers of protection, abundance, healing, and love. It is a magnificent source of nutrients, antioxidants, minerals, and fiber. The enzyme bromelain inherent in pineapple aids digestion and fights inflammation, and topically exfoliates by breaking down dead skin cells.

**Pink tourmaline** This feminine pink stone activates the heart chakra, brings forth feelings of peace, love, support and comfort, as it eases anxiety and promotes good cheer.

**Plum** Deeply hued plums are rich in antioxidants, vitamins, minerals that beautify and support good health. They are ruled by Venus and carry the magick of beauty, love, sex, and protection.

**Pomegranate** Pomegranates are great bringers of money, while their abundance of juicy seeds denote their creative and fertility magick. They symbolize the blood of life, and therefore have a special place in youthful beauty potions, both internal and topical. They help strengthen the proteins that form collagen and elastin, and are rich in fatty acids that lock moisture in and keep debris out. Rich in vitamin C, they stimulate collagen and can lighten age spots.

**Pumpkin/pumpkin seed extract** The classic symbol of autumn, beloved pumpkin is a beauty superstar. It bursts with high levels of vitamins, minerals, antioxidants, and essential fatty acids—not to mention healing and money magick. Lunar-ruled, it soothes, protects, and hydrates while its vitamin C and zinc content increases firmness. It's an excellent choice for sensitive and acne-prone skin.

**Raspberry/raspberry seed** Loaded with antioxidants and vitamin E, raspberry seed prevents the destruction of skin cells, wards off premature aging, and helps to maintain water balance in skin. It is healing to eczema and psoriasis, and protects against UV damage. Ruled by Venus and water, it brings forth happiness, love, and protection.

**Rose absolute/attar/rosewater** Though the rose appears delicate, it is actually one of the oldest symbols of strength. A flower of Venus, and sacred to both Freya and Hathor, it has been revered for its beauty magick, as well as that of love, luck, divination, healing, protection, and enhancing psychic abilities. Rose is active, yet soothing, targeting fine lines and wrinkles with a variety of vitamins, minerals, and antioxidants. The difference between attar and absolute is the extraction process, which leaves the absolute with a stronger scent due to chemical or alcohol solvents, and is therefore more often used in perfumes. The attar is steam-extracted, making it a purer choice for skincare.

**Rosehip** A gift of Venus, this superior moisturizing oil is extracted from the hidden fruit of the rose once the petals have fallen away. Easily penetrating into the skin, it hydrates and moisturizes without causing breakouts or clogging. It boasts a natural retinol in the form of beta carotene from vitamin A to promote cellular turnover, repairs tissue and builds new tissue deep within the skin to support firmness. Rosehips also contain high levels of vitamin C, stimulating new collagen and repairing skin while protecting against UV damage, making them a fabulous choice for elixirs as well as skincare. They possess all the magick of the rose itself, but have a little extra charge of sexuality.

**Rosemary** Interestingly, lusty rosemary is also known as "elf leaf," and bears the properties of love, healing, intellect, and youth. In addition to these palpable gifts, it is also known for its ability to increase cellular metabolism to boost circulation, stimulating not only mystical prowess but bountiful hair growth, and firm skin.

**Ruby** Solar-powered ruby strengthens and nourishes skin with a vibrant, fresh energy. It increases blood circulation, bringing a sunshine glow to your face.

**Sage** Sage in potions is not to be confused with the sage you burn. It is a Piscean culinary herb, beloved for its vibrations of health and longevity. Antioxidant and anti-inflammatory, it detoxifies and heals skin while imparting moisture. It is also known to reduce swelling and improve the appearance of stretch marks.

**Saffron** These sensual, solar threads gift us with their heady aroma, depth of flavor, and lots of bright, sunny happiness magick. Rich in manganese, saffron promotes glowing skin, along with boosting immunity and easing digestion.

**Sandalwood** Long prized in Ayurvedic traditions, sandalwood is a dear friend to your skin: it fights visible signs of aging, keeps skin clear, and lightens hyperpigmentation. White sandalwood is ruled by the Moon, and has strong properties of healing, protection, and banishing. It exudes the delicious musky scent we associate with the beloved bark; however, red sandalwood is *not* aromatic. Red sandalwood is Venus-ruled and used in love magick. All sandalwood is considered sacred, and endangered. (See Resources p. 235.)

**Sapphire** Ruled by water, sapphire has been used for centuries to impart hydration to the skin. It carries the vibration of love and purity, while restoring and rejuvenating the skin. It also helps to protect against environmental stresses.

**Saw palmetto** The extract of this petite palm tree is used to prevent hair loss, reduce inflammation, ease migraines and improve men's health. It is said to give the male libido quite a boost!

**Schisandra berry** A prized adaptogen in Traditional Chinese medicine (TCM,) schisandra is valued for its ability to harmonize the body. It balances hormones, supports the brain, liver, kidneys, and digestion. It is also known as a great beauty tonic, allowing the skin to retain moisture and firmness while promoting shiny, healthy hair.

**Skullcap** A member of the mint family, skullcap has long been used to quell anxiety. Mildly sedative, it promotes relaxation, and magickally promotes love, peace, and fidelity.

**Shea butter** A highly moisturizing fat, shea butter is also antibacterial, making it a great crème base for all skin types. Rich in antioxidants, it promotes cell turnover, helps fade stretch marks, prevents dandruff, and heals skin. *Shea butter is derived from a tree nut, but it does not carry enough of the proteins that cause allergic reactions, so most people find it a safe choice.*

**Shungite** Purifying, cleansing, and detoxifying, shungite is also highly protective, both emotionally and psychically—with an added benefit of protecting from electro-magnetic fields (EMF's) transmitted by electronic devices.

**Smoked alderwood salt** Also known as *salish,* this is created by slowly smoking the salt over wood, usually Alder, one of the sacred Celtic trees. Known as the King of the Waters (willow being its Queen,) the Alder grows in the faerie realm, where land and waters meet. It attracts powers of self-protection, divination, and healing.

**Smoky quartz** Gorgeous, earthy smoky quartz connects you to your root chakra, clearing to allow energy to flow freely. This grants openness around sex, so you can fully enjoy it!

**Snow lotus mushroom powder** Also known as tremella, snow lotus is a superfood mushroom that hydrates amazingly, both internally and topically. It penetrates skin easily, helps to maintain moisture levels, and assists in cell regeneration. Ruled by earth, mushrooms gift the magick of strength and heightened psychic awareness.

**Spinach** One of the ultimate green beauty foods, the pretty leaves of spinach are overflowing with vitamins, minerals and micronutrients. Magickally, you can't beat it either—ruled by the cosmic luck-bringer Jupiter, it draws money and abundance to you in a *big* way.

**Spirulina** An auspicious partner to chlorella, spirulina is also an excellent source of clean plant protein, loaded with antioxidants and nutrients. It supports collagen production, smooths fine lines (while helping to prevent new ones!) and carries the magick of water. Purchasing a chlorella/spirulina blend makes it easy to enjoy the combination benefits (See Resources p. 235.)

**Star anise** A celestially-shaped powerhouse long associated with aiding psychic awareness and bringing luck, it also does *wonders* for your skin. Potent, fragrant compounds help to reduce the appearance of wrinkles while firming and repairing damaged skin, simultaneously keeping breakouts at bay.

**St. John's wort** A classic anti-depressant herb, St. John's Wort also does wonders for skin. It soothes, hydrates, and protects, and heals both irritations and scrapes. Ruled by fire, this solar-powered plant is used in magick to ward off illness, impart strength and protection, and bring forth love and happiness.

**Strawberry** This gorgeous offering of Venus brings you glowing skin! It balances, nourishes, and fortifies with abundant vitamin C—well known for its collagen production prowess. Strawberries are pure pleasure in every way, including the love and beauty magic they are known for.

**Sunflower** The energy of the sunflower is one of exuberant life force. Solar-powered and fertile, sunflower grants wisdom, joy, and good health. Rich in linoleic acid, it helps to build and maintain a healthy skin barrier, which thins as we age. This light, non-clogging oil contains vitamin E which prevents damage to skin cells and protects from UV rays, preventing wrinkles while nourishing with vitamins A, C, and D.

**Sunstone** High-energy, fiery sunstone helps to clear all energies and chakras. It carries potent vibrations, and is used to empower, bestow confidence, increase vitality, give courage, and encourage independence. It also brings good fortune.

**Stevia** Originally hailing from South America, stevia has become a common sugar alternative. It is a natural, plant-derived sweetener with a zero glycemic index and has no calories. Available as a liquid or in powdered form, stevia is very sweet— you only need a small amount.

**Sweet almond** Another oil which moisturizes without clogging the skin is the vitamin E-charged sweet almond. It is an excellent one to mix with some heavier oils, to create a beautiful texture and broad-spectrum beauty benefits, most notably repairing collagen, preventing moisture loss, and lightening troublesome dark spots and circles. It gives the magick of healing while attracting money and abundance.

**Sweet orange/orange** These magick trees aid in release of trauma, and bring clarity to emotions. Solar-ruled, their fruits hold purifying fire magic. These bright lights are fortified with vitamin C and beta-carotene for some serious wrinkle-fighting protection. Added bonus: their cheerful scent is a guaranteed mood-booster.

**Tea tree** This Aboriginal healing plant has long been used to heal as an anti-inflammatory, antimicrobial, antifungal topical treatment. It effectively cleanses and fights germs while easing skin irritations, and is excellent for acne-prone or oily skin.

**Tequila** Mexico's favorite tequila comes from the blue agave plant, which gives this spirit the powers of agavins, a sugar that cleanses the colon. *Pure* tequila aids digestion, contains probiotics, and actually won't spike blood sugar.

**Thyme** Another revered Venusian witches herb, thyme possesses the magic of love, psychic awareness, purification, healing powers, and courage. These scented sprigs are potent both in their energy and their health benefits. Believe it or not, their tiny leaves hold an enormous amount of nutrients, including a saucy measure of iron! A bit of this will fortify the beautifying power of your potions and delay the signs of aging.

**Turmeric** Closely related to that other power root, ginger, turmeric contains medicinal compounds. Antioxidant and anti-inflammatory, this gorgeously-colored ancient spice cleanses from within to keep skin clear and calm, and does wonders for rashes and eruptions. Magickally purifying, it is even known to keep negative energies away.

**Valerian** Watery, feminine valerian root is ruled by Venus, carrying not only her love magick but also that of sleep, cleansing, and protection. Indeed, it is known for all these properties as a staple of practical magick. Use valerian to reduce anxiety, calm nerves, promote restful sleep, and protect.

**Vanilla** This delightful vine wafts in sensually by way of Venus, heavy on the love and sexual magick. It's heady aroma and flavor intoxicates, and its aphrodisiac powers are legendary. Vanilla is also rich in copper, which helps to promote collagen and elastic production. It soothes, protects from environmental stresses, and carries an enchanted scent.

**Vegetable glycerin** A natural, inexpensive humectant, vegetable glycerin attracts moisture. Like all humectants, though, it requires an occlusive (moisture barrier) to make it effective. Combine it with oils like olive, avocado, or butters such as cacao or shea for potent potions.

**Vodka** With its antiseptic and disinfectant prowess, vodka can be effectively used as a sanitizer. When consumed (in moderation, of course) vodka can help with arthritic conditions and hypertension, acting both as an anti-inflammatory and in boosting blood circulation.

**Violet** Lovely violet brings forth love, luck, wishes granted, peace, and protection. It is also a strong anti-inflammatory and skin healer. Fresh flowers are gorgeous, but the dried leaf is a totally acceptable substitute, and will be easier to find year-round. But do plant some!

**Vitamin C powder (ascorbic acid)** Adding this to your topical potions promotes collagen production, protects from environmental stresses (including UV rays,) lightens hyperpigmentation, and firms skin. It is important to use pure ascorbic acid, as the molecule needs to be small enough to be absorbed through the skin. Make sure to keep it (and potions made with it) stored away from heat, light, and air, though, as these factors will cause it to be unstable.

**Vitamin E** A supreme skin loving healer that repairs damaged skin—*this includes wrinkles*—and bestows beautifying fats. Available in bottles and capsules, vitamin E oil has a thick, sticky consistency that takes a little while to absorb into the skin, but is entirely worth it. Pair it with more easily absorbed oils (like jojoba) when you're in a hurry.

**Watermelon** Sacred to Yemanja, lunar watermelon is a beauty food wonder: made of 92% water, it's quite literally drenched in hydration, not to mention nutrients. Blessed with antioxidants and amino acids, it also contains high levels of vitamins A, B, and C.

**White clay** While most clays draw impurities from the skin, white clay holds the distinction of depositing nutrients very effectively. As such, it makes a nice addition to all kinds of facial masques, but particularly for balancing an already strong cleansing or exfoliating potion.

**White peony root** Used in ancient eastern medicine for boosting the immune system, harmonizing the body, and elevating mood, white peony also brightens complexion and wards off the visible signs of aging. Peony is ruled by fire and has powerful protection magick.

**White willow bark** From several varieties of the magickal willow tree comes the herbal remedy often used in place of aspirin. It is believed to be gentler on the stomach, too, than its drugstore counterpart. The best part? It carries the feminine, lunar vibration of the willow, bringing love, protection, prophecy, and healing.

**Wine** Though we think of wine as being purely Bacchanalian, in ancient Mesopotamia twelve vases of wine were offered to the goddess Ishtar every single day. Filled with antioxidants, wine wards off illness, is anti-inflammatory, and is said to increase longevity. Red wine is the solar counterpart to lunar white wine.

**Yarrow** Protective yarrow grants courage, increases psychic ability, and attracts love. It allows us to relax fully, encouraging restful sleep and prophetic dreams. Use caution if taken internally, as it is considered a very potent sedative.

**Ylang-ylang** Sweetly seductive, the dew of the ylang-ylang flower is a tropical treat which enhances mood while fighting wrinkles and fine lines with strong antioxidant powers. It works well as a moisturizing oil for all skin types, promoting new cell growth and improving elasticity. It is also a beautiful natural conditioner that strengthens hair.

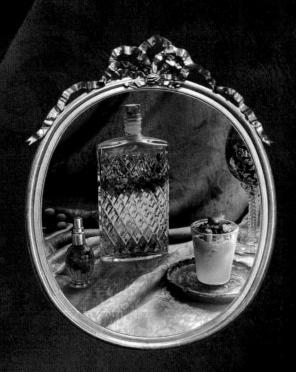

# Resources

Here are some of my most trusted online sources for clean, cruelty-free, well-sourced ingredients and cosmetics. New ones seem to be popping up every day, which I encourage you to try (and I will too!) but I can tell you that I personally go to these companies regularly, and can trust their consistent standards. They also all have lovely customer service reps that can help answer any questions.

# Herbs, Flowers, Oils, Extracts, Powders

―•▶▸•◀◂•―

## Mountain Rose Herbs

One of my favorites, especially for dried flowers and butters.

https://mountainroseherbs.com

## Bulk Apothecary

My main source for base oils, butters, and clays.

https://www.bulkapothecary.com

## Longevity Warehouse

Superfood and superherb emporium for hard-to-find ingredients.

https://longevitywarehouse.com

## Frontier Co-op

Excellent source for the bulk herbs and spices often found in your local health food store.

https://www.frontiercoop.com

## Sunfood

Another great source of powders and supplements, as well as superfoods.

https://www.sunfood.com

## Sun Potion

They carry hard-to-find ingredients, like Lion's Mane mushroom powder.

https://www.sunpotion.com

RESOURCES

## Dragon Herbs

Specializing in Traditional Chinese medicine tonic herbals.

https://www.dragonherbs.com

## Hybrid Herbs

More tonic herbs and a good source for organic Snow Lotus (Tremella) powder.

https://www.hybridherbs.com

## Nativas Organics

I love their potent berry powders!

https://navitasorganics.com

## Banyan Botanicals

Specializing in Ayurvedic herbs.

https://www.banyanbotanicals.com

# Essential Oils

## DoTerra

High quality, therapeutic-grade essential oils.

https://www.doterra.com

## Original Swiss Aromatics

Full catalog of hard-to-find essential oils and absolutes.

https://www.originalswissaromatics.com

# Nail Lacquer

## Zoya

Every possible shade you can imagine, but do get the base and topcoat so they last longer.

https://www.zoya.com

## Butter London

A rich lacquer for a slightly longer-lasting polish. They also carry makeup.

https://www.butterlondon.com

# Makeup

## Ilia

I'm a big fan of their liquid eyeliner!

https://iliabeauty.com

## Thrive Causemetics

A portion of every purchase goes to supporting women and their communities. And their Liquid Lash Extension mascara is a must-try!

https://thrivecausemetics.com

## Acti-Labs

Beautiful eyeshadow palettes, and very well priced.

https://www.acti-labs.com

## Jouer

Their concealer does wonders for my sleepless eyes!

https://www.jouercosmetics.com

## Le Rouge Francais

Lightweight, beautiful lipsticks—a bit pricey, but they come in refillable, eco-friendly, biodegradable cases!

https://lerougefrancais.com

## Addictive Cosmetics

I can't get enough of their matte lipsticks—and they offer sample sizes that make great travel companions when handbag space is at a premium.

https://www.addictivecosmetics.com

# Accessories

## Seek Bamboo

An excellent source for sustainable makeup pads, hair/body/tooth brushes … even dental floss!

https://seekbamboo.com

## Last Object

Washable cotton swabs in an eco-friendly storage case, plus washable makeup pads.

https://lastobject.com

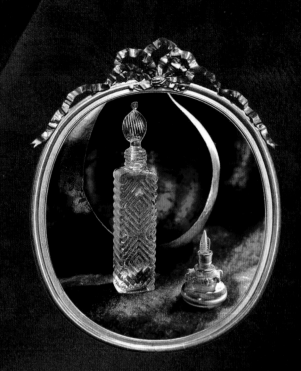

# Recommended Reading

Antol, Marie Nadine. *Healing Teas.* New York: Penguin, 1996.

Ber, Leonid, and Karolyn A. Gazella. *Activate Your Immune System.* Green Bay, WI: IMPAKT, 1998.

Butler, Simone. *Moon Power: Lunar Rituals To Activate Your inner Goddess.* Beverly, MA: Quarto, 2017.

Collins, Elise Marie. *Chakra Tonics: Essential Elixirs For The Mind, Body, and Spirit.* York Beach, ME: Conari, 2006.

Conway, D. J. *Moon Magick: Myth & Magic, Crafts & Recipes, Rituals & Spells.* St. Paul, MN: Llewellyn, 1995.

Cunningham, Donna. *Astrology and Spiritual Development*. San Rafael, CA: 1988.

———. *The Moon In Your Life: Being A Lunar Type In A Solar World*. York Beach, ME: Weiser, 1996.

Cunningham, Scott. *Cunningham's Encyclopedia of Magical Herbs*. St. Paul, MN: Llewellyn, 1985.

———. *The Complete Book of Incense, Oils and Brews*. St. Paul, MN: Llewellyn, 1989.

———. *Magical Aromatherapy: The Power of Scent*. Woodbury, MN: Llewellyn, 1989.

Chopra, Deepak. *What Are You Hungry For?* New York: Harmony/Random House, 2013.

Cousins, Gabriel. *Spiritual Nutrition*. Berkeley, CA: North Atlantic, 1986.

Falconi, Dina. *Earthly Bodies and Heavenly Hair*. Woodstock, NY: Ceres, 1998.

Flynn, Beverly Ann. *Astrology and Weight Control: The Jupiter/Pluto Connection*. Epping, NH: Starcrafts, 2003.

Garrison, Omar V. *Medical Astrology*. New Hyde Park (NY): University, 1971.

Gladstar, Rosemary. *Herbs For Natural Beauty*: Storey; New Edition, 2014.

Hawke, Elen. *Praise To The Moon: Magic And Myth of The Lunar Cycle*. St. Paul, MN: Llewellyn, 2003.

Jansky, Robert Carl. *Astrology, Nutrition & Health*. Atglen, PA: Schiffer, 1977.

Mazzeo, Tilar J. *The Widow Cliquot*. New York: Harper, 2008.

Scoble, Gretchen and Ann Field. *The Meaning of Herbs: Myth, Language, and Lore*. San Francisco: Chronicle, 2001.

Schulman, Martin. *Karmic Astrology, Vols. 1 & 2*. York Beach, ME: Weiser, 1977.

Shaw, Ava. *Your Astrological Guide To Fitness*. Bedford, MA: Mills & Sanderson, 1987.

Simms, Maria Kay. *Moon Tides and Soul Passages*. Exeter, NH: Starcrafts, 2004.

Spiller, Jan. *Astrology for the Soul*. New York: Bantam, 1997.

Snyder, Kimberly, CN. *The Beauty Detox Solution*. Ontario: Harlequin, 2011.

Stevens, Jon. *The Astrology Diet*. North Hollywood, CA: Freedom-Life, 1985.

Wolfe, David. *Eating for Beauty*. San Diego: Maul Brothers, 2003.

Wolfe, David and R. A. Gaulthier. *The Beauty Diet: Unlock The Five Secrets of Ageless Beauty From The Inside Out*. New York: Harper Collins, 2018.